Living in the Dead Zone:
Janis Joplin and Jim Morrison

by

Gerald A. Faris and Ralph M. Faris

Living in the Dead Zone: Janis Joplin and Jim Morrison

By

Gerald A. Faris and Ralph M. Faris

Previously published under ISBN 158500-185-6

Printed and distributed by BookMasters, Inc.
2541 Ashland Road, Mansfield, Ohio 44905.

Canadian Cataloguing in Publication Data

Faris, Gerald A., 1937 -
        Living in the dead zone
        Includes bibliographical references.
        ISBN 1-55212-378-2
        1.   Joplin, Janis. 2. Morrsion, Jim, 1943 – 1971
        2.   Rock musicians – United States – Biography
        I.   Faris, Ralph M., 1945 -   II. Title
        ML420.J77F22   2000   782.432166' 092 ' 273   C00 910639 –1

Acknowledgements

Our work here has been the result of the dedicated enthusiasm of many people, especially those who frequently read our manuscript. So as not to praise the blame worthy, nor blame the praise worthy, as the Greek Sophist, Gorgias, argued, we wish to thank all thos who supported in word and deed the writing of our work.

They include our wives, Susan and Janie, and our children, Lisa, John, and David G. (also responsible for the design of the book's cover), Jason, and David M. They enthusiastically embraced our project, never complaining, always suggesting. The love and support of our families sustained us through the four years we needed to finish this work.

We are especially grateful to Rima Brauer, MD. The purpose of this book—understanding the experience of patients—was advanced by her brilliant, penetrating insights into the intrapsychic complexities of the human mind.

Other readers whose advice proved invaluable were neighbors and colleagues: Tom McNamara, Steven and Susan Wolfson, Graham Gibbard, Sheryl Bedingfield, Anna Follis, Marie Furmanski, Amy Evangelisto, and Martin Spear. Mike Guidice rendered the drawings of Janis and Jim in therapy as well as in the beginning of the first chapter.

We alone are responsible for any and all errors.

Acknowledgments

Table of Contents

Living in the Dead Zone:
Janis Joplin and Jim Morrison

Foreword

The Connecticut Turnpike stretched well ahead of us on that warm spring day as my brother and I drove to a family reunion in Massachusetts. It would be another two and half hours before we would arrive at my cousin's impressive home, a former convent that is now the headquarters for all important Faris family gatherings. I reached for the radio dial, hoping to find some relief from the broken white lines that marked the turnpike lanes, when a voice cried out, singing a melody that instantly carried us back to the 1960s, to the anti-war sentiments that filled the airways, to the epic struggle for civil rights, to the generation of flower children and the music they embraced so passionately. Janis Joplin was singing, and our journey was made ever so much more enjoyable, filled as it was with the memories that "Me and Bobby McGee" so quickly rekindled.

As it turned out, we had unknowingly discovered a "golden oldie" station, so our two hundred mile journey led to inevitable reminiscing, to the tales we tell each other about what happened in our lives when Lyndon Johnson and Richard Nixon were president, when baseball's Mets were finally top dogs, and Vietnam was our major concern. We reminded each other how awful were the clothes we once wore and the conflicts we had; but the music, oh that music, how intoxicating it was! All that from a song recorded almost thirty years ago.

As the music ended, we both remarked how young Janis was when she died, how her death was followed by that of Jim Morrison, also in the prime of his life. I let my mind wander back to the 1960s and the deaths of two very talented performers whose music helped me to survive while leading a platoon of soldiers through the jungles of Vietnam.

Aware that I was emotionally surfing the sixties, my brother, speaking casually but knowledgeably about their deaths, said "They were tragic figures, struggling with a complicated psychiatric condition known as a borderline disorder, ya know," he calmly offered. "I've seen many patients just like them." "Borderline?" I asked, "What do you mean, borderline?" He was referring to borderline personality disorders, to highly distraught and tormented people whose affliction is now very well documented in the clinical literature. I was rather surprised by his confident voice, and asked him to explain why he was so certain that Janis and Jim were borderline personalities. For the next hour he offered me the insights he had gained through intense exchanges with his "borderline" patients, from the wealth of research and clinical case studies, and from the information about Janis and Jim discovered in their excellent biographies and other books detailing their everyday behaviors.

So that was it, I thought. Two masterful, charismatic but deeply disturbed artists died because at the time the basis for their tormented and self-destructive behaviors was not known; no one could help them because there was no help—not unlike the people who at one time died of pneumonia because there were no antibiotics. Worse still: my brother remarked that there are many, many undiagnosed borderline personalities who will remain so because many clinicians, even now, aren't adequately trained to identify such a disorder. In addition, many people are misdiagnosed as having a borderline condition because many clinicians are poorly trained to understand the difference between borderline disorders and other disorders, such as manic-depressive disorder, major depressive disorders and childhood-based post-traumatic stress disorder. He suggested that a more compelling kind of story might be useful in alerting therapists to symptoms that have been associated with the disorder. And that might just help to identify and treat patients who suffer from the same disorder that eventually killed Janis and Jim.

Acting on that conversation, my brother and I initially considered developing a "manual" of sorts that might be useful to therapists and clinicians. Later, however, as our interest in Janis and Jim intensified, we found ourselves entranced by the circumstances of their lives and by the dramatically oppositional and unpredictably volatile nature of the borderline disorder that afflicted them. We decided to dedicate our book to a wider, more popular audience, one comprised of those who loved and appreciated their music when they were alive, and those who still find a deep connection with their music almost thirty years after their deaths.

After all, we thought, shouldn't their fans, who were and are thrilled by their performances but saddened and mystified by their early, tragic deaths be offered insight into the inner core that powered their compelling and often haunting lyrics and music? Convinced of their fans' enduring interest, we constructed this post-1960s social-psychological analysis of Janis Joplin and Jim Morrison.

(RMF)

Preface

No two people captured the imagination and emotions of the "sixties" generation more than Janis Joplin and Jim Morrison. Their dramatic stories have been told in numerous biographies, in film, and in their music. They entered a social arena during a decade characterized by radical social movements, widespread rebellion, and popular unrest. The distant but deadly southeast Asian war and the historic struggle of civil rights groups afforded Janis and Jim the opportunity to generate extraordinary psychedelic sonatas aimed directly at the dissatisfied, the alienated, and the young. Their early deaths increased the passion felt by their fans, spurred numerous films, internet web pages and biographies. Their characters and deaths also guaranteed a consistently high demand for their music, now technologically enhanced, that endures even among those too young to have experienced the tumult of the sixties.

Almost thirty years after their tragic deaths a persistent fascination with their lives remains intact. New biographies exploring the life and times of Janis and Jim were published in 1990, 1991, 1992 and 1993. New releases of their recordings are planned or are already released. Films of their concerts and interviews are stocked in video stores. Younger generations of Americans are intrigued by the music of Janis and Jim if not by the aura surrounding their deaths. *Newsweek* (7/15/93) reported that during the first six months of 1993 more than 500,000 Doors records and over 200,000 Joplin albums were sold.

Conversations about Janis and Jim evoke positive and highly emotional responses. One young sales clerk told us she absolutely loved and adored Jim Morrison, while wrinkling her nose at Janis Joplin. Another, noticing that we were purchasing a Joplin tape, volunteered exuberantly, "She's great, she's super", and asked us if we had read Myra Friedman's *Buried Alive.* People in their forties who remember Janis and Jim and who may have also seen them in concert recall them as incredible, wild, and then usually add approvingly, "crazy." Those under thirty think of the two as fantastic and legendary free spirits whose lives ended tragically.

Why then this book? A number of excellent biographies on Janis and Jim have been published. Filmed interviews and documentaries are readily available in video stores along with their music. Their lives have been captured in motion pictures - Janis in a story called *The Rose* and Jim in Oliver Stone's *The Doors.* What new light, then, can we shed on their lives?

All the publicly available information on Janis and Jim is *descriptive,* that is, it describes their behavior, temperament, moods and personalities, and records faithfully the course of their lives and careers. What that information doesn't provide is a reasonable explanation for the dissonant and relentlessly self-destructive behavior that led to their premature deaths. Serious biographers have been compassionate and psychologically perceptive in describing the desperation and torment of each, but have exhibited little interest in or ability to identify the underlying causes of their disorders. And that is not surprising.

Determining causality is understandably complicated and risky when done from a distance. This has not prevented some from engaging in unsupported theorizing and speculating, however. Popular explanatory accounts of their lives reveal less about Janis and Jim than about the authors' lack of familiarity with the dynamics of psychological disorders. These surface level analyses have typically pointed to their abuse of alcohol and drugs as if that were a sufficient explanation by itself. Others blame self-destructive patterns of depression rooted in early family conflicts, traumatic incidents in their lives, or the overwhelming pressures created by fame and stardom. But as we hope to reveal, the root causes of the extended and debilitating despair suffered by these two tragic talents has simply not been established.

This book has come about by chance. We had planned originally to explore the lives of several famous people (Joplin, Morrison, Monroe, Hendrix, Garland and others) for the purpose of uncovering the internal forces responsible for their widely publicized distress. In addition to these "stars," we also intended to examine certain characters from literature and movies. As our research progressed, we became increasingly fascinated with the accounts of the lives of Janis and Jim, experiencing a deep sense of sadness as we learned about their greatly troubled existence. In Janis' case, we were struck by what appeared to be a deeply felt pain, exhibited in news clips, which captured her unrelenting hopelessness. In those clips, she behaves as a child who is alternately angry, charming, confused, and witty while answering questions from reporters. We read of her search for love in an attempt to quiet the internal demons through endless, transient sexual liaisons, wild, partying and alcohol abuse. Like Janis, Jim struggled unsuccessfully for meaning by avoiding or running from a similar feeling of hopelessness. His life too was characterized by the aggressive behaviors, alcoholism, and antics for which he was so well known.

Both presented in public and in private as

highly neurotic and disordered, and as lacking the resources which we all need to soothe ourselves when alone: the ability to make our existence tolerable, to experience satisfaction from relationships, and to possess a sense of ourselves and our continuity. It is this deficit, this missing quality of their inner world, that was at the root of the persistent and debilitating hopelessness they both experienced. That hopelessness is what faces those unfortunate enough to find themselves living in the dead zone—a term frequently used by my patients to describe how their *borderline personality disorder* feels to them (described in detail in the first chapter).

Prologue

I know Janis Joplin. She's been in my office many times. I have seen her funky clothes, heard her cackling laugh, been the target of her good-natured wisecracks, experienced her unpredictable affect storms, and felt her agony. I have lamented the dismal, pitiable quality of her life, wrestled with her demons, and tried to help her with the most intractable of inner conflicts. And I've observed her relentless drive toward self-destruction.

Jim Morrison, too, has been in my office. Like Janis, he was bleeding from self-inflicted wounds. Unlike Janis though, his demeanor was frequently abstruse and enigmatic, his ever present arrogance being the most prominent feature of his interactions with others. He uses words to confuse, attack, and diffuse; yet his demons, like Janis', were unmerciful and in the end did not permit him to escape. Finally he fell victim to them as he slid into the abyss.

Perhaps I should say that I have seen such patients who bear a striking psychological resemblance to Janis and Jim. I have seen these patients in psychiatric hospitals and in my private practice. I have also supervised interns and clinicians who were treating them. Of course, these patients are not exactly like Janis or Jim. No person is ever identical to another—not even an identical twin. People have their own unique combination of traits apart from their pathology, as do my patients. But they are very similar to Janis and Jim in that they engage in the same terrible struggle with the emptiness of the dead zone.

Overcome by constant misery and beset by a vast and dreadful emotional emptiness, these patients are unable to contain the forces that drive their rampant impulsivity. Lacking a stable sense of self and vulnerable to sudden emotional episodes, they desperately seek to sustain unsustainable relationships, as did Janis and Jim. Like them, they lead lives that are both intense and chaotic.

One should not, however, misconstrue the analysis we provide in this book as an attempt to diminish the value of Janis and Jim's creativity nor of their contributions as performing artists. Neither should one take this work to be yet another exposé of the "real" lives of two rock stars. Janis and Jim should not and cannot be defined solely by their affliction; and it is certainly true that their lives, regrettably, have been greatly exploited.

Still, we do wonder how they were able to bring so much energy, creativity and excitement to their music in spite of their affliction. Speculating in that direction might be intriguing, and we do have a few thoughts on the matter as we attempt to understand the psychological roots of their illnesses. We provide explanations of their behavior which are drawn from more recent developments in modern psychiatry and psychology—developments that we believe constitute the most comprehensive account of the disorder that ultimately took their lives.

[GAF]

Jim

There are twenty cemeteries in Paris. In one, Pere LaChaise, are the graves of Chopin, Sarah Bernhardt, Oscar Wilde, Marcel Proust, Gertrude Stein, Isadora Duncan, and Balzac. And Jim Morrison.

The weather was overcast and cool during a visit to Paris in the fall of 1993 when I (GAF) spent a few hours at the cemetery researching this book. The ubiquitous French penchant for decoration and style can be seen at Pere LaChaise, in the well kept, sometimes elaborately designed grave sites, many with small altars inside a larger stone chamber above the ground. On ordinary days, the cemetery is filled with people visiting loved ones. Uncharacteristically, many of the visitors were young, ranging in age from fourteen to twenty-four. They came in large numbers, guided by the notorious but revealing graffiti on the monuments leading to Jim Morrison's grave. All of them, like the weather that day, were somber and solemn, tombstone tourists trekking in seemingly endless numbers, hoping for some kind of emotional experience at the grave of a man who died before they were born.

Uniformed guards have been permanently stationed at Jim Morrison's grave for the past thirty or so years to prevent it from being destroyed piecemeal by visitors. The damage to other gravesites has been so extensive that the French may refuse to renew the lease for Jim's plot (Jim's gravesite at Pere LaChaise was leased, not purchased). Everywhere along the way, the graffiti spray painted on other grave sites reflects the intense feelings that Morrison could elicit. The diverse, often contradictory messages expressed in the graffiti are fascinating. Read perspicaciously, they underscore how his music was interpreted by his fans, by those to whom he expressed his hopes, his conflicts, and his usually disdainful assessment of the human condition. There were many of the symbols from the peace movement of the sixties and 'I love you Jim' with a signature. Others wrote the name or lyrics of some of his songs like "The End" and "Break on Through" as if they were by themselves prophetic. A few with troubled minds wrote things like 'kill parents.'

Many Morrison fans appear reflective, sad, gloomy and/or nettlesome, like Morrison himself, absorbed with existential matters, sex, and death. Much of Morrison's music amplified such concerns, as in "The End," "Five To One," "When the Music's Over" and "Unknown Soldier." Odd and mystifying feelings are expressed in such songs as "People are Strange," "Strange Days" and "I Can't See Your Face In My Mind." He characteristically acted in weird, obnoxious ways on stage — actions that seemed to have had no purpose other than to allow him to dissipate pent up tensions.

I interviewed dozens of these young mourners from Germany, France, Belgium, England, Italy, Austria, and the United States. Without exception, in their mood and manner they revealed a reverence for, and a strong identification with Jim Morrison. These young people derived whatever meaning they needed from the music, poetry, and antics of Jim Morrison's life in order to cope with the conflicts and deep tensions of their own adolescent struggles. Their misreadings of Morrison varied. Some thought of him as a free spirit, others as a rebel with a cause. They knew of his self-destructive behavior but chose to disregard it. He was their hero, no qualifications necessary.

Janis

Janis Joplin is not buried anywhere. In *Buried Alive* Myra Friedman writes that Janis' body was cremated in accordance with her will and her ashes scattered by air along the coastline of Marin County, California. Thus no pilgrimage to a Janis Joplin shrine is possible. Fans have to make do with her music, a documentary film called *Janis,* and a bronze statue of her in several of her well known stage postures located in the Port Arthur Historical Collection at the Lamar University Library in Port Arthur, Texas. Her fans, however, are no less dedicated.

Ask anyone who attended a Joplin concert, and in a flash of memory he or she will return to the scene. One fifty year-old Ph.D. who had seen Janis in concert told me, "It was extraordinary. She had gotten a hold on the deepest passions of the audience. It was an incredible scene. Constant motion, erupting like a volcano, holding nothing back—you had to be there. I'll never forget it."

If you talk to enough fans of the two great singers, you will quickly hear the noticeable difference in the kind of responses elicited from fans of Janis as opposed to Jim's. Joplin fans, like Morrison fans, make of her what they need and see her as sympathetic to the conflicts they feel. But it appears that there is a way to distinguish many of Jim's fans from Janis' fans: different psychological agendas.

Janis' fans give off a softer feeling of exuberance and a "go for the fun of it" attitude. They talk of Janis as a life-loving, good-time girl who wasn't going to be bound by dumb rules, and as one who spoke her mind. Like Janis, her fans are preoccupied with matters of life, hope, love, and sex. One can easily discern these preoccupations in songs such as "Try," "One

Good Man," "Piece of My Heart" and, in general, from her public persona of "Get It While You Can." Thus, it's not stretching the truth to suggest her fans embraced those themes.

The two are alive and well in the songs, antics, and agonies remembered by the many fans today who were inspired by them and felt their conflicts. Increasingly, new CD's and tapes can be found on the shelves of music stores as their music is recycled and updated year after year. Each of these performers possessed a unique quality of style and content, of personality and intensity that appeals to similar audiences. That the music of two deceased rock stars has such a following is not unusual. However, the psychological and emotional elements of the Morrison and Joplin phenomenon that accompanied their music are seldom found today. Even the enthusiasm popularly expressed for Elvis Presley's music has more to do with the nostalgic response of the generation which actually heard the music than it does with deep feelings of emptiness and despair. The Joplin and Morrison phenomenon arises from the more primitive, conflicted elements of psychological development and as a result has the potential to reach an audience that cuts across generations.

We believe there is great irony in the fans' perception of these two stars because much of their behavior was misinterpreted. Fans were encouraged and comforted by Janis and Jim's excesses, by their endless search for thrills, and their rowdy, impatient, attention-seeking, chaotic behavior. In actuality these self-destructive tendencies were symptomatic of something more. Little did fans know that Janis and Jim were two unique, eccentric but talented people experiencing the unrelenting, existential despair that is characteristically found in certain personality types—

personalities destined to live their lives in a constant struggle with the hopelessness of life in the dead zone

Chapter One: Living in the Dead Zone

A mind is not to be changed by place or time.
The mind is its own place, and in itself Can
make a heav'n of hell, a hell of heav'n.
Milton : Paradise Lost

Since the deaths of Janis and Jim, psychologists have developed many promising explanations, complete with technical terms, of that awful place the mind inhabits. Thus, if you consult the appropriate journals you will encounter terms such as "object inconstancy," "object impermanence," "identity disturbance," and "splitting," to name a few. Each term has been used to describe some feature of the environment that patients refer to as the dead zone. All the terms taken together are supposed to offer a complete picture of that experience. But these terms, so carefully developed by clinical psychologists, simply do not do justice to the terrible psychological toll paid by people who experience the emptiness of that zone.   Widely heralded icons of music, Janis and Jim never really knew what the zone was, though they were driven into that dark and foreboding place most of their adult lives.

Imagine a mind teetering on the edge of an unimaginable abyss, a devastating emptiness in which there is no self, no other, and no reference points — a terrifying nothingness, a null point of mind.   While encompassed in the nothingness, the mind experiences a confounding chaos of confusing noise and an indescribable sense of catastrophe. Unable to grasp or comprehend the reality of others, the mind thus cannot comprehend itself. The totality of the experience leaves the sufferer with no "I" feelings, no sense of actually existing, no self-reality. The continuity of self-feelings, moment to moment, is relentlessly broken by the emptiness, the spacelessness, the nothingness.

Imagine next the frantic scrambling for a person or place to provide an unchanging, reliable anchor, a reassuring "rock of Gibraltar" to quiet the noise and fill in the spacelessness so that the mind might perceive its own existence. The mind's hope is to achieve but a modicum of the necessary "I" feeling, of a convincing reality of self. A struggle ensues, a battle begins.

Janis and Jim died not knowing that the hell they endured came from their own minds. A little understood disorder in the 1960s, their affliction engulfed them leaving no way out, no relief. One of the most complicated and disruptive states of being, it is difficult for someone in it to describe and almost impossible for those not there to imagine. But it has been studied and identified, and is now able to be treated with modest success. In clinical practice, it is currently known as **borderline syndrome** or **borderline**

personality disorder. The term 'borderline' is unfortunately confusing. The term initially referred to what was previously understood to be a disparate collection of diagnostic entities such as 'infantile personality,' 'unstable personality,' 'pseudo-neurotic schizophrenia,' and 'borderline schizophrenia' to name a few. A number of clinicians viewed some of these diagnoses as being on the 'borderline of psychosis' while others thought of the diagnoses as actual 'borderland' disturbances. After the research peaked in the sixties and seventies, the term borderline had gained such widespread use that it was difficult to change (even though these patients are not psychotic).

How can we describe Janis and Jim's condition? How can we make their experience of life in the dead zone comprehensible? They experienced one of the most complex and confusing disorders known in clinical psychology, then and now. What do we know about the disorder today that we didn't know when they were alive?

Perhaps we should start with the term most frequently used by patients in therapy to describe that state of mind, that place to which they are driven daily: the dead zone. Even if we had been able to interview Janis and Jim, we would have had great difficulty in obtaining unambiguous and revealing accounts of their tortuous, emotional experiences (And both were widely known to be very bright, articulate personalities). Nonetheless, we offer you a glimpse of that terrible place by tapping into the accounts offered by patients who have been thrust into the dead zone. Our book's title actually came from a patient who wrote that she was:

> . . . always scared and
> empty, like a void. Always
> feeling on edge. Will I

always be like . . .this? I feel so all alone. No matter what, it's like I'm unreal, not here, like the living dead; no, not even dead . . .just . . . nothing.

As is often the case with complex personality disorders, many different descriptive accounts are given. Some patients reject the qualifier "dead" for "zone," preferring instead terms such as intense conflict, or "non-zone." One patient found different metaphors more helpful as she rejected the dead zone imagery altogether:

It is not a zone, because to me that implies a place in which something is, an inexplicable oneness of being and peace. I am both the thing and the space and the time, and nothing comes in or out because there is no out or time or separateness . . . The snow metaphor seems more apt, it is a whiteout.

And, as if to emphasize her objection to the term *dead*, she added:

I wish it were the dead zone because in such a place one could be free of feeling—for that is to me what dead implies—but it is a place void of understanding while full of feeling all the more painful feeling, because it is not capable of dying or ending or stopping or being understood by self or others. But to call it a dead zone is to misidentify it as well as those who inhabit it.

However differently patients may describe their borderline experiences, they experience, as did Janis and Jim, an inner world of feeling that leads to contradictions in their behavior, distorting and frequently destroying their perspective, their relations with others and their sense of well-being. Within them emotional tidal waves known as *affect storms* may rage for hours or days, reappearing and then suddenly disappearing, leaving their most valued friends exhausted, confused, and frustrated.

Because they are unable to control their emotional states for very long, they are controlled by them. Their behaviors consistently reflect this rule-by-chaos phenomenon. Researcher/clinician Marsha Linehan has suggested that people with this disorder "are like people with third degree burns over 90% of their bodies. Lacking emotional skin, they feel agony at the slightest touch or movement."

In *I Hate you – Don't Leave Me*, Kreisman and Straus describe the borderline disorder as "emotional hemophilia; [a borderline patient] lacks the clotting mechanism needed to moderate his spurts of feeling. Stimulate a passion and the borderline emotionally bleeds to death."

That chaotic internal state of mind that characterized the lives of Janis and Jim was relentless and insidious. That they managed under those conditions to produce exciting and cutting edge music is remarkable; that they both died at the peak of their careers and at a very early age is not surprising. They could not have realized that their overwhelming sense of desolation was not a widely shared experience. Janis and Jim dragged themselves through life while tormented by chronic feelings of emptiness, intense loneliness, blankness, and numbness, as if living in a black hole. They were constantly left on the edge of confusion, wracked by intolerable tension, and consumed by alienation and desolation. Generally, borderline patients do what Janis and Jim did. That is, they create chaos and disorder, anger and despair in many if not most aspects of their lives, especially in their relationships.

Like others living in the dead zone, Janis and Jim engaged in behaviors that destroyed many of their interpersonal relations. They shifted quickly from one emotional state to another, continually instigated self-damaging, impulsive actions, and in the process experienced profound and consuming identity conflicts. When asked, Janis and Jim would attempt to justify themselves with a long list of rationalizations such as "I was angry, I'm being mistreated, I want to get it on man, get down, get groovin', I am incensed at injustice, I am just a rebel, I want to live life to the fullest, I was feeling bored, I'm just different and the world can't handle it," and so on, as if these explanations were entirely acceptable excuses for their aberrant behaviors.

The question we raise and answer in this book is whether Janis and Jim, with the help of a therapist, might have been able to assess their mental states more carefully. Might they have come to understand the inner world of feelings and to comprehend the emptiness and dread of their own dead zones? Would they have begun to speak as others have of the dead zone as a *void*, a *nothingness*, a *state of not being*. Might they have been helped? We think so.

Each seemed to have the problem of feeling "out of it", of having to "rewrite" one's history to make sense of one's behavior, because each desperately needed reality to conform to what they were feeling in the moment. Thus personal history or incidents in their past were illegitimately reinterpreted to validate the present. The instability of their own "I" feeling impelled them to seek reassurance of their own existence. Jim Morrison relied on Pamela Courson to reestablish his "I" sense. Janis seemed to rely on family correspondence, audiences, and a number of relationships which could not survive her self-destructive behavior. Both relied on alcohol and heroin to blunt the despair of living in the dead zone.

Janis and Jim, like others in the zone, always appeared to be depressed, though without the longing, the sense of loss and grief characteristic of those who are clinically depressed. Any depression they experienced was merely secondary. Depressed people often have difficulty with appetite, sleep, concentration, and being interested in life, (see Appendix II) while people in the dead zone usually do not (unless they are clinically depressed in addition to being in the dead zone, suggesting multiple diagnoses). Janis and Jim had no identifiable loss or incident to account for any depressed mood and, from all the sources available on their lives, no family history of depression.

Modern clinicians have come to recognize in borderline patients feelings that we believe Janis and Jim continually felt: moodiness, agitation, emptiness and despair. The tragedy is that they could not possibly have won the battle against the disorder, at least not at that time. Clinicians were not yet in a position to offer them relief, so misunderstood was their affliction.

The following are three central characteristics that clinicians today associate with the lives of people living in the dead zone.

1. Intense and chaotic efforts to escape the experience of the dead zone.

Like others suffering from this malady, Janis and Jim tended to create turbulence in their environment, and to act out in various ways by blocking, diffusing, masking or weakening the horrific, emptiness of the dead zone. Unaware of the root causes of their deep anxiety, they often behaved in ways typical of those trying to escape or contain the experience of these feelings. They frequently abused alcohol and drugs, engaged in sexual promiscuity, and behaved in emotionally unstable, dramatic or bizarre ways, to include explosive outbursts. Janis and Jim exhibited many of the personality traits found in varying combinations among people in need of escaping from the dead zone. Often both Janis and Jim could be:

chaotic   childish
cranky   hostile
moody   reckless
seductive   volatile
demanding   extremely unpredictable
unreasonable   intense
mercurial.

The King and Queen of Rock and Roll also displayed some of the following behaviors and symptoms typical of the borderline condition:

outbursts of rage	diffuse anger
panic attacks	acute anxiety
phobias	superficiality
moodiness	detachment
thrill-seeking	sexual escapades
emotional lability	feelings of despair
physical complaints	clinging
anorexia	bulimia
alcohol or drug abuse	withdrawal
inappropriate gestures	emotional detachment
perceptual distortions	suicidal ideation
cognitive distortions	dissociative experiences

Unaware of their affliction, both Janis and Jim engaged in these behaviors in their futile struggle to escape.

2. A disturbance in identity formation or sense of self due to the dead zone.

The process of identity formation is complex. All humans must work through it. The lifelong, chaotic, and pervasive nature of that process in Janis and Jim suggested the borderline condition to us. Janis and Jim, like many borderline patients, had loosely configured selves which were maintained through a career identity, while outside that career their cohesive self-feeling gradually dissolved. In both cases, they found people who become stabilizing figures (husband, wife, boss, parent, friend, mentor, etc.), people who periodically helped them maintain psychic balance. Pamela Courson partially fulfilled that need for Jim, while several people in Janis' life (plus her family via letters from home) helped stabilize Janis to a degree. When these measures failed, each sought additional external props for self-containment, such as drugs, alcohol, sex, intense relationships, and other active distractions. There was a kind of surrender to the impoverishment of the inner world in Jim, resulting in a profound withdrawal from experiencing or feeling anything (as revealed, for example, by his retreat to France). The late psychoanalyst Erik Erikson's, term 'alienation' applies to most patients with the disorder. They try to isolate themselves from all the intolerable experiences of an internal emptiness and a disordered self by walling off all feelings. We think that this is how Jim must have felt at the end of his life. Others become resigned to the painful feelings of despair and develop a blank self, a numbing of all feeling experience except at a superficial level, giving others the impression of a shallow and peculiar personality. Janis on the other hand, was apparently struggling to survive even as she took that fatal dose of too-pure heroin and alcohol.

3. An incapacity to maintain stable, intimate relationships.

Our analysis points to the lives of Janis and Jim as revealing a clear pattern of *unstable, shifting relationships* with frequent, unpredictable alterations in emotional attachment or detachment. They appeared to lose personal boundaries while exhibiting such behaviors as clinging, avoiding, demanding, manipulating, or some combination of these. Their behaviors became increasingly Jekyl and Hyde-like, with sudden changes in mood, from being amiable and relaxed to mildly irritable or overtly hostile, as though they were trying to provoke a fight or some other extreme reaction from others. For some in the dead zone, a kind of consuming, primitive hunger develops, making it possible for others to sexually or emotionally enslave them. These patients manifest a desperate need for emotional relatedness complicated by a deeply felt intolerance for the frustrations inevitable in relationships.

Janis and Jim were caught up with the fear of abandonment, envelopment, or disappointment (otherwise known among clinicians as the "need-fear" dilemma). Like many with this condition, Janis and Jim often used people and things as "transitional" soothing objects like teddy bears or other toys. The person or thing selected may have no real existence of his/her own, but may exist only to gratify the individual's needs and reduce the tension created by this condition. For Janis and Jim, these relationships were usually symbiotic, dependent, narcissistic, or exploitative, and were not mutually gratifying or satisfying.

The Core of the Disturbance

The essence of the disturbance is currently being clarified by clinical concepts emerging from psychoanalytic research such as *splitting* and *object constancy*. Hoping to avoid making our discussion too technical, we will refer to *splitting* as a weakness in a person's ability to integrate the different sides of himself or different sides of others into one complex whole personality. Thus, to Janis and Jim, the same spouse or lover appeared to be ever shifting in his or her essence: one day good, helpful and gratifying, the next day hostile, frustrating and rejecting.

The differing and sometimes contradictory sides we all possess are experienced by the person in the dead zone as separate and distinct personalities, though not in the sense that the term schizoid connotes. It is as though the friend or spouse is not the same person all the time and cannot be trusted, is not reliable or consistent. Such a misperception of a constantly changing interpersonal environment leaves the patient vulnerable to high anxiety, anger, black/white thinking, inconsistency, confusion, erratic functioning, and defensiveness.

Object constancy is the ability of patients to access internal images of important people in their lives, and/or to have feelings about those images. Developed early in childhood, possession of this ability allows one to feel connected to others, to feel real and to be able to soothe oneself. In contrast, patients living in the dead zone have poor object constancy, understood as having no people (images or representations) to access or relate to. That's precisely why they feel so empty and desperately alone – and so would any of us under those conditions.

The consequences of splitting and object inconstancy are also revealed in other areas of life such as work or school, where one's capacity to focus and perform is crucial. Despite being highly intelligent, Janice and Jim were academically inconsistent and remarkably unproductive, revealing a failure to engage in any sustained intellectual effort in these settings. They were unable to organize their mental resources for an extended period toward any goal requiring intellectual persistence and discipline. For example, they often experienced great disparities in school or in interpersonal exchanges, good work performance but chaotic personal relations, good sexual functioning but poor personal relations. While Janis and Jim could be utterly amazing in concert, they were unable to function consistently within and between the various domains of daily life (education, career, and interpersonal relations).

Dead zone inhabitants can be somewhat primitive at times. Clinicians also talk of them as *unintegrated*. They are strongly inclined to the instantaneous present, so that when difficulties arise in important personal relationships they become revisionists (they remember things poorly). A multitude of good experiences in a relationship can be quickly forgotten in the context of some real or imagined but trivial slight by the partner, spouse, lover, or friend. Jim's outrageously stormy and volatile love/hate relationship with Pamela Courson is one good example. His many abuses of that relationship and his frequent angry exchanges with her led to his detachment from her. This usually resulted in emotional confusion, acting out and uncontrollable drinking (Jim almost always drank to get drunk), followed by episodes of anxiousness and then quiet reconciliation. Always on alert status and lacking a sense of proportion in private matters, Janis and Jim possessed precious little capacity to absorb softer feelings, the softer feelings needed to soothe themselves.

Though the criteria cited above are generally useful in recognizing the disorder that took the lives of both Janis and Jim, the condition was only just beginning to be understood in the late sixties and seventies. Complicating the matter, many people who are experiencing the dead zone are not moody or affectively disruptive in most settings outside their most intimate relationship. (Some can function very well at very high levels. The character played by Glenn Close in the movie, *Fatal Attraction,* is a good example of the efficiently functioning professional who becomes unraveled when she is intimately involved.) It was another decade before clinicians became sufficiently familiar with these patterns to offer effective treatment. Therefore, no one was really in a position to recognize the disorder while Janis and Jim were alive.

The Common Elements Of The Dead Zone

Two dimensions can be employed to organize the confusing information about the dead zone in order to identify the more common features and escape the distraction of variations in behavior and personality. We have chosen to present the common elements of the disorder as succinctly as possible with two over-arching dimensions as a guide. In doing so, we hope to avoid discouraging the reader by rendering descriptions that are too technical or otherwise confusing. One dimension is the *level of functioning* and the other is the *emotive vs. the detached* dimension.

Level of functioning refers to how well such individuals can maintain themselves in a work or education environment, how well they can present themselves in the social milieu, how well they can engage in human relations, and how well they can contain the ordinary stresses of life without a deterioration in their reality testing. For example, higher level individuals with this condition, living in more safe, structured environments with support systems and reasonably collaborative partners, will most likely have better social relations and more resistance to slippage in reality testing under stress than lower level ones. The more severely disordered individuals will be more vulnerable to breakdowns requiring hospitalization. They will have more chaotic relationships or none, and will eventually manifest more of the non-specific symptoms. These include symptoms such as erratic and unstable patterns of behavior, less tolerance for anxiety, more acting out to relieve inner tension, more clinging, more highly dependent and ambivalent relationships, greater fear of abandonment, panic attacks, greater impulsivity, increased likelihood of dissociative experiences, anorexia, bulimia, alcoholism and drug abuse. Viewing the lives of Janis and Jim with this newly constructed criterion, it is our judgment that they functioned at a *moderate* level of disorder.

The **emotive vs. detached** dimension refers to the differences among individuals in the degree of emotional expression and communication. On the one hand, highly *emotive* types, like Janis, may *act out* whenever they feel any of the inner tension associated with life in the dead zone. They often create chaotic turbulence in the environment while expressing neediness and demanding attention. On the other hand, *detached* types do not so readily exhibit emotional lability (except under stress), seem to keep more to themselves, and frequently appear to be more distant. Jim appears to have possessed characteristics of both types, withdrawn and alone for long periods of time, followed by emotionally engaged episodes in which he created great turbulence. Despite his episodes of impulsivity, he was just as likely to seek resolution of the same inner conflicts and tensions associated with life in the dead zone by an emotional withdrawal and avoidance of real relationships. In Jim's case, though his behavior appeared more controlled at times, he was *detached* from any true connection to others, habitually engaging in transient, superficial relationships bereft of emotional investment.

Psychoanalyst W. W. Meissner has conceptualized these "emotive vs detached" types as constituting what he calls a "hysterical - schizoid spectrum" or continuum, placing Janis on the hysterical end and Jim on the schizoid end. He has further unscrambled some of the confusion resulting from the wide differences in outward behavior among people on this continuum by describing them in terms of the higher order, middle and lower order personality functioning described above (Meissner 1984, chp. 1). Thus we can now think of these disorders as having degrees of disturbance from severe through moderate to mild. We can also think of some of them as having degrees of emotionality, attachment, and outward turbulence, ranging from high to low. What this means for us is that people living in the dead zone present a number of complex behaviors, exhibiting the symptoms of the disorder to various degrees and through a variety of characteristics.

People with this condition have a long history of mild to moderate symptoms and atypical or unusual behaviors beginning in childhood or early adolescence (though many of the problem behaviors are also common to several other psychological conditions). They do not all manifest the same degree of acting-out behavior, paranoid tendencies, narcissistic traits, overt emotionality, hostility, antisocial attitudes, and vulnerability to drugs and alcohol. Nevertheless there are certain observable behavior patterns, signs, and symptoms that are common to this condition, transcending the confusing differences in personality style and nonspecific signs and symptoms.

Chapter Two: Janis And Jim—Popular Accounts And Misconceptions

From childhood's hour I have
not been as others were.
I have not seen as others saw.
                    "Alone" by Edgar Allen Poe

By most accounts, they were the king and queen of rock and roll in the sixties, and both died at age twenty-seven due to the abuse they had visited upon themselves. A generation heard Morrison's call to "break on through" and Joplin's cry that "you know you've got it if it makes you feel good." When an interviewer asked Janis what she thought young people wanted she replied, "sincerity and a good time." There is no record of any Jim Morrison answer to such a question, but we can be reasonably sure (based on biographical information available to us) it would have been esoteric and dark.

They were both born around the same time to conventional, white southern families. Both were very intelligent, given to outrageous behaviors in high

19

school, and rejected by most of their classmates. Both were narcissistic, rebellious, anti-authoritarian, and intensely needy, and they exhibited severely conflicted inner selves. While Morrison was seen as an unpredictable Jekyll and Hyde, Joplin had much more of a go-for-broke, roller coaster-like unpredictability. They knew each other, liked each other's work, and were lovers for a while.

All the biographical accounts report that they once met at a party, which was noteworthy only because Janis ended up slugging Jim on the head with a whiskey bottle for behaving in his typically obnoxious way. Neither initially sought fame or even the status of a rock singer. They simply hung out with the boys. Neither could contain their constant disruptive impulses or maintain any kind of mature, mutually satisfying, non-manipulative or non-abusive intimate relationship. As we will show, both were consumed by the relentless inner desolateness of the dead zone. Both abused drugs and alcohol throughout their adult lives and engaged in endless rounds of chaotic relationships that left much emotional debris in their wakes. Sadly, the best adjectives we can think of to describe the progress of their lives is self-destructive and anarchic.

The similarities go further. Both Janis and Jim were highly intelligent with clearly superior IQ's. Despite a maverick status in school, each read and absorbed quality literature and had a natural proficiency with language. According to his biographers, Riordan and Prochnicky (1991), Morrison had a recorded IQ of 149. Janis's superior intelligence was manifested in verbal skills, a quick wit, and a familiarity with good literature. One has only to watch those engaging interviews in the documentary "Janis" to confirm her mental agility in give and take situations, and her latent intellectual capacity.

Jim also read extensively on many dark and arcane subjects, wrote poems of arguably publishable quality, and struggled with existential issues both in verbal and written form through his music and writings. He and Janis were both multi-talented. A precocious child, Janis frequently demonstrated above average ability in art and drawing, and later in vocalizing and interpreting music, composing songs spontaneously off the top of her head. Jim's writings and poems are surreal and quite obscure, but clearly authored with intelligence and intense feeling by one with an obvious talent for vocalizing and writing songs. Each had an electric effect on their audiences that has rarely been matched in intensity and in longevity. People who have been to a Joplin or Morrison concert recall the experience with amazing clarity and enthusiasm thirty years later.

What was not widely known, however, is that both suffered greatly from a highly disorganized emotional life. This rather uncommon disorganization is experienced by many as an emptiness which leaves them without the capacity to take in and feel the soothing that comes from early attachments to others as previously mentioned. It is a despair that is felt every waking moment by those who unintentionally find themselves struggling with the necessity of living a life in this emotional black hole.

Popular Misconceptions

The pathos of their lives and the tragedy of their deaths invites a kind of easy speculation about causes. Relatives, biographers, and fans have considered the possibilities and offered their speculations, which generally fall into one or more of the following hypotheses.

The first is that the subculture of substance abuse destroyed them, that Janis and Jim were overtaken by the fast-paced excitement and demands of rock star life. Drug and alcohol abuse were so pervasively a part of that life that they were inexorably drawn in and became what would be called today chemically dependent, a condition from which they were unable to escape. Each died from either a drug overdose or from a lethal combination of drugs and alcohol.

That other great talents who performed in this era also died under similar circumstance is a matter of historical record: Jimi Hendrix, Elvis Presley, Marilyn Monroe, Judy Garland and John Belushi. In April 1994, Kurt Cobain, lead singer for the group *Nirvana,* killed himself with a shotgun blast after years of drug abuse. His suicide came only a few months after River Phoenix died from complications of a drug overdose. We will not be surprised to see these celebrity tragedies continue.

The public knowledge of and attitude toward drugs was different in the sixties. The counterculture to which Janis and Jim belonged encouraged the use of drugs to liberate one from stultifying convention and to "expand one's mind." This was a time when gurus such as Timothy Leary recommended the use of mind altering drugs such as LSD, and when the medical profession for the most part ignored the extensive use of amphetamines by film stars, apparently acquiescing to the demands of a subculture that would not be denied any pleasure or experience.

On this line, then, performing artists, musicians, and other creative people frequently indulged in drugs and alcohol abuse, a widely accepted and understood feature of their environment (though the effects were not fully understood). Can the trajectory of the lives of Janis and Jim be explained by pointing to their chemical dependence on drugs and alcohol, moving them so quickly into the self-destructive behaviors that eventually killed them?

It is perhaps easier to understand why this hypothesis has so many proponents than why it is, nonetheless, a misconception about the two. The list of drug-related deaths among entertainers is long, and the use of drugs for relief of stress by many show business people has a well documented history. When we note the more casual attitude toward drug use during the sixties—the general ignorance about the addictive nature of some drugs and the popular practice of combining drugs—the likelihood of being "caught up" in the drug scene becomes a compelling and believable idea.

However, this hypothesis raises more questions than it answers. For instance, what of the well-documented feelings of alienation and despair both Janis and Jim repeatedly voiced long before drugs and alcohol became so pervasive in their lives? If one takes the view then that the ingrained drug culture of the entertainment world pushed Janis and Jim into their graves, how can we account for their distressing behaviors when drugs or alcohol were not involved? The problem here is that any causal connection we make between the substance abuse and their notorious behavior must account for the periods when they weren't using drugs or alcohol and yet continued to exhibit the same impulsive, crude, and self-destructive behaviors. Under these circumstances, to posit a cause and effect relation between the abuse and their self-destructive behavior is simply wrong.

A second problem with this hypothesis is that it

does not account for the fact that these two people engaged in self-destructive behaviors when they were adolescents. According to their biographers, who provide lengthy accounts of the childhood and adolescent behaviors of Janis and Jim, their early behaviors were very much like those of their adult years. One need not be a clinician to recognize the presence of an emotional disorder after reading of Janis' teenage excesses in Myra Friedman's biography, *Buried Alive*, or in *Love, Janis*, a book by Janis' sister, Laura. According to Jim's biographers, this pattern held for him as well. No matter how detrimental drugs and alcohol later became in their lives, it would be incorrect to assume that alcohol and drug abuse were anything but symptoms of something else, i.e., symptoms of a deeper, less obvious disturbance.

There are still other details of their lives which disconfirm this hypothesis. Despite the publicity that is given to the drug-related death of a star, the vast majority of performing artists do not die so early in their lives, nor do they engage in chaotic, self-destructive behaviors — though many might have had some experiences with drugs and alcohol. Elvis Presley and Jimi Hendrix for example, for all their abuse of various substances, did not exhibit such persistent and aggressive, chaotic behaviors. Nor did they verbalize the feelings of alienation and despair that were so characteristic of Janis and Jim. Again, it is quite clear that drugs and alcohol may have complicated the lives of these two great personalities, but cannot alone explain their tragic lives.

A second hypothesis has to do with the idea that Janis and Jim were essentially stable personalities and that fame and fortune had a destructive effect on their egos with neither able to handle the pressure. On this line, then, the vicissitudes of fame and fortune rather than alcohol and drug abuse are offered as the cause. One fifties movie, *A Face In The Crowd*, (in which Andy Griffith played a decent and conventional guy who was corrupted by a sudden rise to fame) is a not so subtle dramatization of the perils of show business success. Those who propose this account wish us to believe that success in that competitively cruel and aggressive world of entertainment is actually a defeat for one's spiritual and emotional health. Especially important in this view is the idea that the star is continually exploited and increasingly alienated, finally turning to drugs and alcohol for relief. This theme is encountered in at least one biography of Marilyn Monroe, and is suggested in the movie based on Janis's life, *The Rose*. Thus either their egos are artificially pumped up from the fantastic rush and adoration of fans — setting them up for a fall — or they are manipulated and dehumanized by agents or directors so that they become exhausted and demoralized.

It is taken as a given that the temptations of "big" money, the carnal pleasures and the fame and casual lifestyle of show business can ruin the hardiest of souls, and that the exploitation of Janis and Jim was so intense that it should not come as a surprise that their lives ended so. A rather widely held hypothesis, it does have a degree of validity, though perhaps only the appearance of respectability. The high divorce rates for big stars as well as their highly publicized use of drugs and alcohol offer support for this view.

Under close scrutiny, however, this popular speculation fails to make the required connection between the lifestyle and the deterioration in the performer's psychological health and general well being. The impressions gained from headline stories notwithstanding, the overwhelming majority of successful stars and show business people who are presumably subjected to the same pressures do not become self-destructive, do not live chaotic public and private lives and do not die of drug overdoses. Janis and Jim experienced no more show business pressure than others who reached the same level of success. We emphasize this fact in spite of the great publicity given to the deaths of a *seemingly* large number of famous rock and Hollywood stars: Elvis, Hendrix, Monroe, Garland, Belushi, Kurt Cobain and so on. These deaths aside, many other stars had to cope with the pressures of stardom that were a constant source of aggravation in their lives, but which did not *cause* the inner conflicts that eventually destroyed them. Thus we must look further into the personalities themselves for the answers.

A third hypothesis may be summarized as follows: Great but tragic stars may have experienced something terrible in their backgrounds, some trauma or particular family disturbance that shaped their personalities in ways leading to tragedy. This hypothesis is based on the critical Freudian/psychoanalytic perspective that "the child is the father of the man," and that what happens to a child during the developing years directly and indirectly determines the characteristics of the adult. For Janis, the speculation is that she had a cold and rigid mother and an unsympathetic family, that she was stifled and not allowed to be herself by hostile peers, forced to accept the parochial values of a conservative, religious southern town in the "suffocating" fifties. Her acting out behaviors are seen as a reactive search for her real self and a desire to be free and to be loved. In Jim's case, a particularly gruesome auto accident witnessed early in his childhood would provide the explanatory variable for his premature death when combined with a family characterization similar to Janis'. It is regrettable, insist the proponents of this hypothesis, that they were unable to overcome those difficult "background" hindrances and were thus consumed by them. Speculations of this kind are written daily when reports of school shootings or other dramatic and destructive acts are committed by individuals. Apparently we have a difficult time looking at behaviors as signs or symptoms of some larger problem, while accepting the "something happened back there" explanation at face value.

Were Janis and Jim's childhood experiences responsible for their destruction? Were mom and/or dad too punitive, too rigid, too unavailable, too conventional, too controlling, too unemotional, too conflicted or too - (fill in the rest with your views on parental failures)? Were there traumatic experiences?

Based on the wealth of good data from recorded interviews with both Janis and Jim, from the many biographies, and from anecdotal reports, this hypothesis is simply insupportable. To begin with, no record or anecdotal report has ever been found which supports the idea that either was mistreated as a child, nor is there any claim by Janis or Jim themselves that they were mistreated. In fact, just the opposite is true.

Although her parents could be classified as having conventional values, and perhaps being comfortably middle class, Janis's parents were portrayed by her biographers as tolerant of her attention-seeking, outrageous behaviors, encouraging of her intellectual and artistic interests, and deeply concerned about her well-being. Janis' sister Laura in her 1992 book, *Love Janis,* includes many letters and phone calls from Janis to her mother and family, and convincingly dispels any doubt about the strong bond between them.   The same take about Janis and her family was presented by Myra Friedman twenty years earlier in *Buried Alive*.

That Janis' parents were concerned about her lifestyle and the frequent chemical abuse there is no doubt.   Yet they remained supportive of and responsive to her throughout her life. We know of no biography of Janis that describes her parents as a problem to her in that way, nor of any other account of her life that confirms this glib and popular but mostly faulty hypothesis.   Based on the reliable information currently available about Janis, it has no validity.

The same hypothesis fares no better when considering the life of Jim Morrison. Despite some dramatic conflicts with his parents over "values" and "attitude," and despite an outrageous pattern of misbehavior as a child, his family life was otherwise quite stable.   His parents supported his endeavors and generally tolerated his difficult personality. Though Jim showed early signs of emotional problems—in contrast to Janis who did not—his family was neither hostile toward him nor considered dysfunctional in the conventional use of the term.   His later attitude of hostility toward them is better understood as a consequence of his inner struggle with the dead zone. So while Jim was temperamentally difficult (as was Janis, given the available evidence) we simply cannot attribute his emotional conflicts to a dysfunctional or abusive family.

While speculation about Jim's family is not the basis for explaining his life, other popular accounts focus on a childhood experience he had at the age of four while traveling with his parents in their car. There was reportedly a serious automobile accident, the aftermath of which left the passengers (Navaho Indians) bloodied and suffering greatly. Morrison later verbalized about the accident a great deal and its effect on him. Many have hypothesized that young Jim was traumatized by the incident, affecting his life from that day forward. As a kind of postscript to that hypothesis, it is alleged that his family was lorded over by his father, a naval officer and aircraft carrier commander who was reportedly rigid and controlling.

In *Break On Through,* Riordan and Prochnicky suggest that some people thought that Morrison suffered deep psychological trauma from that incident. They cite the findings of parapsychologists who, after looking into the details of the accident, describe the possibility that Morrison was possessed by the souls of the dying Indians. Morrison frequently described this incident in rich detail, possibly supporting the claim that he was so shaken that he was unable to continue his life in any normal way. His subsequent on-stage Indian Shaman-like dancing appears rooted in this early experience, according to those subscribing to this hypothesis.

But to suppose that he drank to quiet the demons that invaded him at the accident scene, or that he was possessed by the souls of the dead, is to engage in nothing more than a highly speculative exercise aimed at understanding Jim's life and death by looking to supernatural explanations. This account, of course, is completely unwarranted. Why don't others who experience a particularly gruesome accident exhibit the peculiar behaviors and antics that characterized Jim's life? Methodologically, the evidence for the hypothesis of early childhood trauma does not support a connection between the incident and his disorder. The hypothesis represents bad science in that selective episodes from his childhood are used in an ad hoc and post hoc manner to account for his disturbing and self-defeating behaviors.

Finally, a more recent hypothesis, emerging from the increasing recognition of the prevalence of depressive disorders in the general population, suggests that Janis and Jim suffered from undiagnosed major depression. The alcohol and drug abuse that so characterized their desperate lives is seen as a consequence of this untreated clinical condition. This hypothesis, while certainly explaining the suicides of many public figures, does not fit Janis or Jim. Neither had exhibited the basic symptoms of a major depression such as constant fatigue or loss of energy, diminished ability to think or concentrate, an overtly depressed mood and markedly diminished interest or pleasure in most activities most of the time. (See Appendix II for complete list). One who is depressed experiences life with apathy, strains to carry on with life, is usually consumed with feelings of guilt or self-reproach and a sense of loss and longing.

Using these as significant criteria, we would be hard pressed to claim that either Janis or Jim suffered from depression. In fact, to any of their close friends and relatives, nothing was further from the truth about their lives. Additionally, none of their biographers has ever suggested depression. Therefore that hypothesis cannot offer a plausible account of their mutual misery anymore than the previous two hypotheses could.

What then can we say about these highly popularized and glib accounts of the causes of Janis and Jim's self-destructive lives? Methodologically flawed, extravagantly speculative, often at odds with reputable evidence, and marked by rudimentary applications of modern clinical diagnostic categories, such "explanations" should be easily dismissed. Regrettably, they have persisted for far too long. We now have available to us more substantial explanations such as those drawn from enriched descriptive categories rooted in what clinicians now term *borderline disorders.*

We take it to be a major concern of this book to describe Janis and Jim by applying the current clinical understandings of these disorders in order to offer revealing accounts of what actually happened to them. The advances of psychology and psychiatry over the past thirty or so years since the deaths of Janis and Jim provide us with a qualitatively different picture of the two. If they had been exposed to the benefit of therapy rooted in these recent insights, both might have survived. Our hope now is that others so afflicted may be diagnosed and treated in a more timely manner.

Chapter Three: Janis Joplin, A Woman Left Lonely

> Take another little piece of my heart now
> baby, You know you've got it, if it makes
> you feel good . . . .

Perhaps no modern figure embodied the characteristic features of the borderline personality or was more familiar with the experience of the dead zone than Janis Joplin. Remarkably extravagant, often witty and crude, highly emotional yet creative and intelligent, she affords us now, some thirty years after her death, the opportunity to perform a psychological postmortem. While we hope to demonstrate that she could easily be diagnosed today as having a borderline condition, we also hope to reveal that she was more than the sum of her anarchic frames of mind.

Whether in biographies reviewing her life or in documentary film interviews with her, Janis consistently presents as a high energy, extremely talented, sharply humorous personality. The life of Janis Joplin is described in all her exuberance in *Buried Alive*, by Myra Friedman. In it we are presented with an extraordinary portrait "written with a sympathetic intelligence, and at times a fiercely lyrical voice" according to Time magazine. Friedman's account is astonishing and revealing, as are the actual interviews with Janis shown in the documentary *Janis.* An interested analyst will find a dazzling array of the symptomatic features now associated with borderline personalities.

In *Janis,* the film producers captured a smiling, wisecracking, hopelessly unintegrated, anxious, very lonely woman who sang with that overwhelmingly powerful and emotionally breathtaking voice; one who had a cackling laugh, who dressed outlandishly in feathers and a boa (like Bessie Smith, one of Janis' heroines) and who had a propensity to overuse sixties' slang such as *cat, man, dude and right on momma.* She was indeed the Janis we had imagined after reading *Buried Alive.*

As our research into her life progressed, we were as much fascinated as educated, in that our interest in understanding and evaluating her began to engender a growing sense of sadness and empathy for the torment she endured. We became more engrossed in the powerful emotional forces expressed in her singing. Friends of ours who had once seen Janis in concert recall her electrifying performance: the music, the audience reaction, the shock to the system and the explosion of emotional energy that filled everyone with wild abandonment. Afterward, the intense feelings aroused were followed by a "washed out" effect. Listening to Janis sing, it was difficult to believe the claim made by some who knew her very early, that her voice was fuller and more powerful before she became famous.

In the same film documentary Janis was interviewed a number of times — once on *The Dick*

Cavett Show, later at a reunion in her home town, and while on a European tour. On the Cavett show she was clearly in top form, trading wisecracks and easily outclassing the dapper Cavett in repartee. Friedman writes of a later appearance in which it was clear that Janis was losing her struggle with those dark inner forces over which she had so little control. Subsequent interviews with her exposed an underlying fragility, that of a confused little girl valiantly trying to maintain a crumbling psychologic balance by adopting the extremes of the sixties' counterculture for support.

In our effort to reconstruct Janis' psychology, we necessarily turned to her talented and thorough biographers, two of whom had lived with her (Laura Joplin, Myra Friedman), and to films of her performances and interviews. In addition, we extrapolated from the reactions of those people old enough to have seen her in concert and from the exclamations of her many current young fans who know her only through her reissued music. From the vantage point of the clinician, however, Janis sounded and acted like many patients who have also felt the terrible desolation of an impossibly underpopulated inner world.

How can we comprehend the life of this intense young woman, uniquely talented but consumed by such extreme emotions and a self-destructive capacity? How can the pathos of her life be understood? What accounts for her excesses, her drug and alcohol abuse, and her irrational behaviors?

Was she really any different from the numerous artists, writers, rock stars and political figures who self-destructed, such as Jimi Hendrix, Elvis Presley, John Belushi, Marilyn Monroe, Sylvia Plath, Ernest Hemingway, James Forrestal, Vince Foster, River Phoenix and Kurt Cobain? To respond to that question we must examine the many details of her life, seeking to explain her state of mind as she coped with feelings most of us will never experience.

Background

According to her biographers, Janis Joplin was born to a proper, middle class, bible belt family in Port Arthur, Texas in 1943. In *Pearl: The Obsessions and Passions of Janis Joplin* (1992), Ellis Amburn (1992) describes Mrs. Joplin as conventional but bright woman, a bit of a maverick in her own right, and musically talented.

Laura Joplin writes that her mother was an energetic, musical, attentive mother, always a creative parent, always interested in teaching her children. Mrs. Joplin bought Janis a piano and taught her how to play. She exposed all her children to music, gourmet cooking, artistic and creative activities. She also engaged in many traditional pursuits such as preparing holiday feasts, baking cookies, and making Christmas decorations. Laura Joplin describes her mother as the best teacher she ever knew, insisting that learning from her was a daily experience.

Mrs. Joplin was the organizer of her children's daily lives, a creative spirit who taught her children songs and generally inspired them to learn. Janis' parents were more philosophically liberal than the Port Arthur community, but generally observed its conventional standards. All the major biographers describe the presence of a loving relationship between mother and daughter in spite of Janis's excesses and outrageous adolescent behavior. Janis frequently telephoned her mother during her performing years, seeking reassurance and maintaining contact.

Janis' biographers all point to the strong and loving attachment she had to her father. He was a fun loving, intelligent man who was well loved by his children and who truly loved them. A playful engineer and tinkerer, Mr. Joplin created unusual swings, seesaws, and toys for his kids. Like his wife, he valued thinking and learning, always encouraging the children to participate in dinner table discussions on books, music, and ideas.

He managed to find creative activities for his children even in the limited cultural environment of Port Arthur. For example, he would take them to the post office to look at the wanted posters and to the library where he would advise them about reading material. Laura Joplin recounts how he:

> . . . was especially ingenious at getting the gang of kids to help with the chores. Like Tom Sawyer trying to get the fence painted, he invited everyone over to help wax the oak floors. He cleaned out the living room and dining room and spread the floor with wax. Then he took any number of dirty bare feet and strapped clean towels on them. Off he would send us to skate and play bumper cars on the glass-like surface the new wax created. We never had so much fun. (Joplin 1992, 32)

Laura Joplin noted that her parents were very concerned about Janis' tendency to react so negatively to community values and standards. As a result she was often subjected to hate and ridicule. Although the Joplin family was apparently more liberal than the community (with respect to civil rights for example) they managed to conform to local norms whenever they didn't seriously conflict with their liberal core values. They cajoled, lectured, and finally set limits on Janis' strange behaviors in an effort to help her fit in. "Please don't set the world against you," Janis was often advised. When all else failed they sent her to a counselor and even considered family therapy at one point.

Based on the many accounts, letters and interviews available since Janis's death, it is difficult to escape the conclusion that she came from a stable, secure, and emotionally supportive family, and that her early childhood years at least were peaceful and happy. We conclude this despite the continued dissemination of the notion that Janis had a damaging childhood which caused her loneliness and despair. And there is still more to learn from her biographers who all corroborate the details of her family life.

From Myra Friedman, Laura Joplin, and Ellis Amburn, we learn that Janis was a shy child, cooperative and easy to raise, cheerful and very normal. Janis' mother is quoted as saying that as a child Janis did exceptional school work, was accelerated in the third grade, had no behavior difficulties, and never did anything deserving correction. Remarking once that Janis did need more attention than other children, however, her mother described her as rather "unhappy and unsatisfied without it." Otherwise in interviews with her biographers, Janis consistently recalled her childhood as nearly idyllic.

Janis' adolescence, however, received no such label. She once remarked, "then the whole world turned, it just turned on me". According to Amburn, Janis became unpopular in high school, a wallflower early on, not very pretty, and plagued by an overweight condition and serious acne. She developed a bad reputation because she could be outrageous and provocative, acting-out and engaging in wild, unusual, and strange behaviors throughout her high school years. She would later become the first "beatnik" in that unappreciative town. Janis had a "foul mouth", ran with others so inclined, expected to get her own way, and would try anything. Some called her a "slut" and "pig," often throwing pennies at her as a sign of disrespect. By the time she arrived at junior high school, Janis was belligerent, frequently expressing her ideas in a strident voice while showing off her abrasive and alienating lifestyle. She was also astonishingly naive, gullible, and impressionable (Amburn 1992, 14).

Frequently narcissistic, stubborn, thrill-seeking, and trashy, her activities at age fourteen would be diagnosed today as *conduct disordered.* The hallmarks of the disorder in Janis included impulsivity, erratic behavior, oppositionality, and emotional reactivity coupled with early promiscuity. She was unpredictable, hung out with hoodlums, often took dangerous risks, and even showed up drunk for graduation. Amburn felt that "something underlying in Janis put her in destructive situations" (Amburn 1992, 1-35). Not simply rebellious, Janis craved acceptance, had a great need to exhibit herself, and had almost no control over her impulses as she got older. She read voluminously, had a strong mind and intellect, was talented in art and music, and had a kind heart. Yet she never lived up to her potential.

While a senior in high school, she managed to insert herself into a sophisticated group of very talented male musicians, becoming "one of the boys." After graduation, Janis fooled around, drinking and having fun. Shortly thereafter she spent some time in a psychiatric hospital for a condition she later alluded to as a nervous breakdown. She rose to fame during that rather peculiar historical period known as the turbulent sixties, a time when many were intent on loosening the moral and political rigidities of an earlier era. Rebellious and irreverent, the major countercultural figures from that decade exerted such an irresistible pull on her that she soon found a home among people championing the emerging forces of change in San Francisco's Haight-Ashbury neighborhood.

In that milieu, Janis continued to live on the edge and while there, to create a life of artistic excitement, incessant turbulence and chaos. One should not be surprised that she completely embraced the subculture of "sex, drugs and rock and roll." Friedman writes, "attending her concerts nwas like mainlining an aphrodisiac right through the spine." It was in that unalterably "wired" environment that Janis attempted to engage life, hoping to find the feeling she could not experience in the dead zone. Perhaps best expressed in her song "Try," she persistently sought what she had been unable to feel. She often said she wouldn't sing any song she didn't feel, that she made no separation between her professional and personal life. Clearly Janis remained hopeful longer than most who find themselves residents of the dead zone; the themes of her songs revealed how desperately she searched for the way out.

Trying Just A Little Bit Harder: Living In The Dead Zone

Tryuh, oh yeah, tryuh, oh yeah
Just a little bit harder . . . .

Janis' biographers all provide rich descriptive accounts of the effects that drugs and alcohol had on her, and of how tumultuous and disordered her life became in the process. Accurately describing how drug abuse can dull the senses, Janis' sister wrote that "it appeals to people with an unquenchable inner turmoil (Joplin 1992). All Janis wanted was "dope, any dope, to smoke dope, take dope, lick dope, suck dope, fuck dope" (Friedman 1992, 48). She also noticed that her sister "was never interested in psychedelics . . . since psychedelics only intensify experience." Asked by a friend once why she did dope, Janis replied "I just want a little fucking peace, man" (Friedman 1992, 49). One might ask, "Peace from what?" The evidence we have collected supports the theory that she sought peace from the unrelenting dread known only to those whose perceptions of life are distorted by a lens focused only on the very edge of existence.

It is important here to distinguish the account of Janis' drug and alcohol use provided by her sister and biographers and accepted by many of her followers from the deeper explanation we offer in this book. A proper diagnosis of her condition requires the separation of symptom from cause as in any psychological evaluation. It is more consistent with the wealth of information available that the depressive reactions Janis experienced after and between concerts were mainly symptomatic of a kind of battle fatigue suffered in her tragic war against the constant sense of emptiness she felt. To substantiate that claim, we must first examine the accounts of her heroin use, beginning with her sister Laura's version.

Janis, Laura noted, reversed the standard practice of most heroin abusers by using heroin *after* the thrill of a successful concert. Speculating that Janis wasn't trying to escape the psychological pain of life circumstances, Laura Joplin suggests instead that Janis was using heroin to avoid the depression which often follows the high of supercharged concerts, much the way a speed freak would smooth re-entry into daily life. To say the least, Janis' performances were always emotionally intense, never failing to move the audience to the apex of arousal. In her sister's view, Janis' heroin use was meant to help ease her way down from the adrenaline high stimulated by her performances, to facilitate emotional movement from the hysterical high of the stage to a normal level of everyday living (Joplin 1992).

It is now conventionally understood that Janis' reliance on heroin for the reason suggested by her sister might appear to be plausible and sustainable. However, that view at best only obscures Janis' emotional condition at the time. While many entertainers require a cooling down period after performances, much as a runner does after a race, most don't employ drugs to do so, nor do many require ingesting both drugs and alcohol in the amounts Janis did. In addition, after the concerts are over, one isn't likely to find such entertainers continually using the two as intensely as Janis did, unless one is prepared to lengthen substantially the calming down time. Or, to put this differently, one should be able to observe Janis during a calm period following the use of drugs, and yet that doesn't appear to be characteristic of her in her after performance binges.

Like so many patients who experience the "incoherent dread" every waking moment, Janis too would try anything to fill her emptiness with the energy of life she derived from frenetic, uncontrolled interaction with those around her. One might easily be exhausted and overwhelmed by the intensity of the hour-by-hour struggle of her daily life. Her unpredictable shifts in mood, thrill-seeking behavior, persistent alcohol and drug abuse, lack of impulse control, sexual obsessions, and emotionally powerful performances in concert were mostly futile efforts at escape, not from depression, but from the "private madness" to which she was driven by that inevitable inner deadness that encompassed her.

We believe that Janis took heroin or alcohol after concerts because they numbed the senses, helping to mask her awareness of the returning torment of emptiness, of the void that attacked her spirit and ultimately sapped her will to live. She did not suffer from depression except perhaps secondarily. Typically depressive people who use drugs look for a lift, a mood elevator like cocaine, or stimulants like amphetamines, not heroin. Rather it was the emptiness hidden beneath the speedy and hypnotic action of a Janis Joplin concert that had to be managed later by "sex, drugs and rock and roll." Her post-concert drug use was no different from her behaviors at any other time she had to face the terrifying experiences of her own inner world.

Her need to manage the nightmare of the void within, a terrifying loneliness unknown and unfathomable to most, also explains Janis' incessant thrill-seeking, absurd sexual posturing, and sexual adventurism. Janis was forever talking about, bragging about or seeking sexual activity. Films of her singing and talking to the audience and filmed interviews in which she frequently makes crude sexual references and asides such as "getting it" and "doing it" appear to confirm this judgment. Many of her most outrageous behaviors and eccentricities appear (retrospectively after thirty years of clinical discoveries and experiences) to have been aspects of her basic personality which also served to deflect, diminish and deter the demons of the dead zone

Myra Friedman was Janis' principal biographer,

companion and friend. She wrote the most psychologically sophisticated, penetrating and emotionally wrenching account of Janis' life. Friedman described one exchange with an increasingly fragmented Janis who expressed that it wasn't "in the cards" for her to have better relationships, that she was doomed to experience only transient and therefore unfulfilling interactions. Disagreeing and pointing out the many opportunities Janis had, Friedman heard Janis reply sadly, "Well, I know, but I get so lonely and it seems like I'm driven and I don't know, I just do things and I don't know why" (Friedman 1973, 56). Most clinicians familiar with patients living in the dead zone, however, do know why, though we have only recently come to understand the special agony Janis experienced. Perhaps she felt most alive and free of her torment only in the rapture of her highly energized concert frenzy. It seems to be no coincidence that she chose singing as her creative and most direct vehicle to express through her body and breath the torment within.

Searching For Love: Me And Bobby McGee

From a clinical perspective, Janis' preoccupation with sex can easily be explained as her attempt to "manage the dread", and as subsequently revealing the difficulty she had with what psychoanalysts call "object relations."

Read how Friedman describes this phenomenon, albeit in a less technical way:

> Janis was consumed and driven by a need for love that was preposterous in its magnitude, her excessive narcissism the result of bitter frustrations and the very

stuff of her insecurity, her desire for constant attention and her gluttonous hunger for approval. She was fanatical in pursuit of affection while rendered incapable, by the self-direction of her feelings, of establishing intimate relationships. Like a longing child crying for love, her aim was to receive, to take into herself a comforting warmth of which, for whatever reasons, she felt acutely deprived. With an obsessive and insatiable need such as that, what sex would fill it became a secondary matter and the physical demonstration of affection a substitute gratification for what she essentially craved. (Friedman 1973, 61)

Later, Friedman expands on her explanation for Janis' crude, overt sexual behavior on stage and everywhere and the bravado exaggerations of her sexual escapades:

But Janis breathed, thought, felt, acted at a primitive level that was nearly absolute. Even in her twenties, she was still like a hurt and pleading child who wants exactly that very love complete in the physical embrace, and sex, in a way, was a valid synonym for what she was in search of. (Friedman 1973, 125)

We take this account to be another example of the desperate search for the "love," a search for missing internal objects, i.e., mental "representations" of the essential people we all must have stored in us to feel "real," secure, filled up, and soothed. It is nothing less than the search for the primitive mother, the mother of infancy who could calm all anxieties and bring the soothing that the child cannot bring to itself. Without the capacity to develop and hold on to these internal representations of the mother, the child is left totally alone in an empty internal world, to struggle interminably with a relentless "object hunger" that cannot be satisfied. Again, Friedman is quite helpful in capturing what love meant for Janis:

> It wasn't love as an adult knows it: no sharing, no interest, no commitment, no giving, none of those things at all. But it really was love to her. In her hunger for affection, she was nearly amok. Her constant pursuit of physical contact resonated with echoes of infant longing, and frustration of such a need could not help but produce an unbearable anxiety. In that sense, sex was a palliative, an escape from tension that could not be endured, thus making sexual relief of inordinate, overbearing importance. (Friedman 1973, 128)

In part, she was a lost child with talent, who could not sustain any long term, non-exploitative relationship. Her impulsive and provocative actions were efforts to contain and satisfy desperately felt, immature dependency needs. Janis' unbearable anxiety came from her life in the dead zone and it prevented the growth and maturation of her personality so necessary for stable and satisfying object relations. According to Friedman, she tended to experience others as a child would. Her intimate relations would always be unstable, tumultuous and tragically unsatisfying.

Friedman points out how Janis wouldn't sing anything that didn't fit with her feelings. In one interview from the film documentary *Janis*, she tells the interviewer that she did not have a private life different from her performing life. In the first chapter we discussed the term *object relations*, meaning the relationships with people important in early life. An examination of the lyrics that she sang, both her own and those written by others, suggests the clinical concept of a "search for the object," a search doomed to failure because she had no capacity to experience the object (person) in a mutually gratifying way. Even the titles of her songs express deep longing and sorrow:

Try	Ball And Chain
One Good Man	Half Moon
Down On Me	Get It While You Can
Cry	I Need A Man To Love
Piece Of My Heart	A Woman Left Lonely
Bye, Bye Baby	Little Girl Blue
No Reason For Livin	Buried Alive In The Blues
Move Over	Women Is Losers
Me And Bobby McGee	All Is Loneliness

Searching For Janis: Nothing Left To Lose

Another aspect of life in the dead zone is the presence of a markedly distorted or unstable sense of self. Here again Friedman portrays Janis:

> Janis was swamped in her own pizzazz
> and amplification quite apart from a
> word of print or even her stage

performances.   In that bellowing, bouncing, jangling clamor, there were those who saw a 'self.' But Janis was afflicted by an emotional astigmatism. Each second was clear but there was no focus. She was disordered, decentralized and diffused (Friedman 1973, 129).

These insightful observations by Friedman are consistent with the diffuse, anxiety driven actions and experiences of someone who lacks an "inner cohesion" and a stable identity.

Characteristically, those in the dead zone develop a diffused and unfocused self which, in Janis' case, left her struggling to find something at the core of her being, something that might rectify the blurred and unsteady perception of herself. She adopted first one then another identity, either dramatic or symbolic (victim, tough guy, sex queen, party animal, anti-establishment heroine, rock star, and so on). The significant consequence for Janis was a unique kind of intolerable psychic tension.

One example of her quickly shifting identity experiments can be found in her decision to take a new name, "Pearl." The poetic irony of this new identity was not lost on Friedman, who describes Janis' agony by penetrating the surface explanation:

But Pearl was another story, a hard-drinking, swearing, always partying, fuck anybody, get it on, get it off, stay stoned, keep on rocking, floozy, flourishing under the tyranny of an applause that didn't come just from the galleries. And still, lurking like an amorphous ghost behind that public persona, there was another Janis, in that last year asserting herself in equally clear definition, but thriving in an isolation as deeply painful as the most solitary of prison confinements (Friedman 1973, 227).

Finding the "Pearl business just too eerie," Friedman observes that, *"the schism in her personality was quite visible enough, exceeding anything that could be construed as the common contradictions in human nature."* (Italics ours)

If her biographers' descriptions are accurate, Janis had no true sense of herself as a person, woman, or partner. The disturbed self-concept so characteristic of people living in the dead zone, and so well known to experienced clinicians today, left Janis aimless and lost, always seeking to feel that she belonged somewhere. Underlying her insistent claim of uniqueness there was a recognizable person, lost in the confusion.

None of these "identities" gave her what she so desperately needed: a stable, cohesive sense of herself with the capacity to soothe herself and quiet the inner discord. Reflecting the consequences of such disharmony in her sense of self, Janis' relationships were shifting, intense, dramatic, unstable, exploitative, and often confusing to both her and her lovers. These descriptions of Janis are all too familiar to clinicians who work with patients struggling with identity problems.

Sex, Drugs And Rock And Roll: Living For The Moment

Janis' biographers describe her rampant

impulsivity. Friedman's Janis is puzzled by people who "could still maintain some order to their souls."

> For herself, there were only extremes; a world of primitive, unbridled impulses; that, or a realm to police her. She simply could not contain herself without the most rigid of impositions, or so she felt (Friedman 1973, 58).

In 1965, early in her career before fame swept her away, Janis returned home and tried to insert herself back into the tame, conventional community of Port Arthur. By returning to a conventional life, enrolling in a local college, dressing conservatively and attending social activities, Janis hoped the structural constraints of life in Port Arthur would help her gain self control. Friedman believes she was willing to adhere to the norms of Port Arthur because she was petrified of her vulnerability to drugs and frightened of the effects of amphetamines, with their tendency to heighten her awareness of her inner pain. She was terribly anxious then because self-control was such an alien concept to her.

Predictably, Janis found no relief in Port Arthur. While the feelings of dread and inner desolation of those with a borderline condition are often eased by an anchoring structure of some kind and a predictability in their daily lives, they are not eliminated. Tendencies toward self-damaging impulsive actions are powerful and persistent. Sex and drugs are the two most common attractions in this case because they have very intense effects on the nervous system. The effects are in the present moment, soothing, exciting or numbing. They can easily blunt one's awareness and experience of dreadful feelings.

In Janis' case her impulsive urges were only temporarily blocked. After a short period of denial, they inevitably burst forth unbridled, even in environments with external constraints. It is no surprise therefore that a year later Janis left Port Arthur and returned to the life of a performing artist, once again to embrace sex, drugs, and rock and roll.

Later she became widely known to have indiscriminate sex with as many men as she could (and at times with women). The love she sought was neither emotionally mature nor reciprocal. Rather, her sexual liaisons were empty and unsatisfying, leaving Janis continually disappointed and eventually demoralized. Her incessant posturing about finding "a piece of talent" and getting laid was driven by impulses she readily allowed or in fact, could never contain. It is worth noting that although Janis apparently had sexual relations with women, the likelihood is that her sexuality was complicated by the identity disturbance intrinsic to the borderline disorder. This fact must be accounted for by any who try to draw conclusions about her sexual orientation.

This failure of impulse control extended to drugs as well, a fact that is also widely documented. She was unable to resist alcohol, heroin, and barbiturates, though they offered her only temporary relief while leading to her death.

Where's Everybody Going?

> There is no one here at all,
> sometimes not even me.
> I have no thoughts beyond despair,
> No dreams except of death.
> From a poem by a patient living in the dead zone.

In the movie *The Rose*, loosely based on her last years, Janis' character falls to the ground outside a bar and cries out "Where's everybody going?" after her latest boyfriend leaves, fed up with her dramatic boozing and indiscriminate behavior. Here, in that agonizing wail for which Janis was so famous, singer/actress Bette Midler (who in fact knew Janis) captured the poignant torment of Janis' world. It was an empty world without images and representations of people. Without such critical anchors, Janis was left fragile and increasingly unable to stop her downward spiral.

In the light of clinical developments since her death, what is revealed by her need for constant, intense emotions and over-the-top activity is a need to stifle or suppress the dread that lurks just beneath the veneer of everyday living. In some indescribable way Janis must have been aware of her own feeling of deadness, reflected as it was in the despair and unbearable sense of emptiness she experienced in a life without meaning. Though she desperately attempted to fill her life with excitement and distraction, she was never really able to escape the unrelenting nightmare. So Janis was truly a lost soul with a great talent, faced with the impossibility of resolving her need-fear dilemma in intimate relationships, who acted primarily out of desperation. Her tumultuous life was filled with incessant commotion. The sense of herself as an ongoing, continuous and enduring being was absent unless she was engaged in intense, on-the-edge activity. Janis functioned inconsistently, had no center and no focus. Her personal attachments were followed by disregard or hostility. She adopted one, then another dramatic or symbolic identity. None of these identities gave her what she needed: a stable, cohesive sense of herself with the capacity to self-soothe and quiet her inner discord.

Aimless and lost, always seeking the thrill, the next intense experience to assuage the pain generated by eternal feelings of hopelessness and dread, she finally succumbed to the consequences of severe drug and alcohol abuse. Impulse-ridden, wracked by a wretched hunger for human attachments and the inability to be satisfied or soothed by them, lacking any inner sense of being, unable to truly connect with anyone, Janis' agony poured out in that wailing, flailing, tormented voice. We are convinced that part of her hold on audiences had to do with the way the pain in her voice touched some of the existential despair in all of us.

Janis: After All

Janis' experiences in that nightmare are no surprise to clinicians who work with the dramatic, emotional, and empty patient. Based on our current clinical understanding of psychology and personality, we are now able to answer questions that many have asked.

1. What was the matter with her? Why was her life such a chaotic affair?

Based on the information we have gathered for this book from the observations of her biographers, the portrayal of her in films and recorded personal interviews with her, what we have found after all these years may be expressed by pointing to characteristic features of Janis' personality:

- a clear pattern of instability in interpersonal

relationships;

- an unstable and vague self-image and identity;

- shifting and unpredictable moods;

- poor control of impulses and emotions beginning in early adulthood and evident in a variety of contexts;

- a pervasive feeling of emptiness/deadness.

This description happens to be consistent with a well researched, conceptually and empirically established psychiatric diagnosis of **Borderline Personality Disorder** as defined by the *Diagnostic and Statistical Manual of the American Psychiatric Association* (DSMIV, see appendix I) and by the work brilliant clinicians, such as Otto Kernberg, John Gunderson, Roy Grinker, Donald Klein, Robert Knight, and many other psychoanalytic investigators who have described the various characteristics of these personalities over many decades.

In modern clinical terms, the response to the first question is that she was increasingly incapacitated by a type of personality disorder that was little known or understood at that time. Her chaotic life may now be understood as derived from that disorder. In their panic to escape inner feelings of tension and dread, most people with this disorder, like Janis' dramatic example, tend to cut a wide life path filled with debris. (There are also *isolative* types). Many of the people we read about in the daily news and about whom we wonder, "How could they do that?" or "What a stupid thing to do?" or "Why would anyone act that way?" may well be struggling with borderline disorders. And of course the female protagonist played by Glen

Close in the movie *Fatal Attraction* quickly comes to mind as an example of the disorder in the extreme.

We are only now beginning to recognize such behaviors as revealing disorder beneath the surface. It is very possible that many of the violent and destructive interpersonal conflicts between spouses or partners, many drug and alcohol related incidents, many accidents, and many other incomprehensible and socially aberrant behaviors that fill the newspapers everyday are associated with people suffering from various borderline personality disorders.

2. How did she die? Did she kill herself?

We obviously can never know for certain. At that time, Thomas T. Noguchi, M.D., chief medical examiner for the county of Los Angeles found that Janis died of an accidental overdose of heroin, though the presence of alcohol in her blood was also noted. Tests results for other drugs were negative, and the medical examiner found no evidence of violence or foul play. The possibility of suicide was considered and apparently discarded.

As with many public figures who died under unusual circumstances, her death began great speculation as to why and how she died. Some theories are patently absurd and we will not take up space to discuss them—for example that she was killed by the CIA, or by drug lords. But the question remains as to how she died. Was it suicide? Was it really an *accidental* drug overdose?

Both Friedman in *Buried Alive* and Laura Joplin in *Love Janis* were insistent that Janis did not commit suicide, at least not consciously. (Note: Psychoanalytically trained clinicians believe in the paradox of unconsciously intended suicide.) They point to the greater likelihood of a drug interaction between the heroin and alcohol. The possibility of an unintentional overdose of heroin or a dose of heroin too pure for her body are pondered by Friedman. Despite her lifelong struggle with despair, neither Myra Friedman nor Laura Joplin believe that Janis had shown signs of suicidal tendencies immediately prior to her death. In fact, she was excited and ready to record a new song, *Buried Alive in the Blues,* according to Friedman. None of her actions in the 24 hours preceding her death were unusual. The most reasonable explanation for the immediate cause of death seems to be as these two biographers and the Chief Medical Examiner have suggested.

If Janis did not kill herself, but instead was simply another unlucky drug user, then the question as to why she took drugs is pertinent. As we have indicated, she did it to help manage a despair and an unbearable inner tension which were laying waste to her emotional life. If we are correct, her death would not be considered a consciously intentional suicide by any means. Rather it came as a consequence of engaging in behaviors aimed at escaping the barrenness of life in the dead zone.

3. How was she different (if at all) from the many other public figures who died prematurely by their own hand?

It is now safe to assert our belief that there have always been a small number of public figures who have suffered with some form of borderline disorder. Many clinicians believe that Zelda Fitzgerald and Marilyn Monroe are two prominent examples. Monroe was treated for years by the well-known and highly regarded psychoanalyst, Ralph Greenson. Monroe's biographers record chronic behaviors that are consistent with what we know today to be typical of a borderline psychopathology. Public figures like James Forrestal, Ernest Hemingway, Sylvia Plath, Anne Sexton, Bruno Bettleheim, and more recently Vince Foster and Kurt Cobain appear *not* to have been suffering from a borderline condition. Rather they appear to have been suffering from one or another form of undiagnosed depression. All clearly intended to kill themselves. The suspicion now runs deep among clinicians that Elvis Presley, John Belushi and River Phoenix may also have been caught in the psychological trap of dependence on drugs and may or may not have been depressed. They do not appear to have been borderline personalities.

Thus what is clear is that Janis was not like most public figures who intentionally kill themselves due to other disorders that drive them to suicide, such as major depression or bipolar disorder (manic-depression). What is important is that there are few *public* figures who fit the criteria for a borderline condition compared to the larger number of non-public individuals whose lives are tormented by the condition. This seems to be true because in general, a moderate to severe borderline condition makes it difficult for someone to achieve and maintain the public recognition that Janis was successful in cultivating. Janis stands as an exception because of the alchemy of the times, her talent and her disorder.

Chapter Four: Reflections On Destiny: Janis in Therapy

Oh Lord won't you buy me a Mercedes-Benz

The richness and complexity of Janis Joplin's personality are not defined by her emotional disturbance. She was not simply the sum of the parts of the psychopathology described here. Her biographers uniformly describe a vibrant, exciting, instinct-driven, let-it-all-hang-out girl, a woman who was also very intelligent, sensitive and much more. Just how these and other salient characteristics combined with her conflicts to create the original talent that she proved to be is a complicated and little understood process.

Her sexual liaisons were a consuming preoccupation, second only to heroin and alcohol. According to her biographers, they included dozens of men and women of all types including public figures such as Kris Kristofferson (who wrote her biggest hit, *"Me and Bobby McGee"*), Joe Namath, Jimi Hendrix, and Jim Morrison to name a few. For a long time she continued a public relationship with the Hell's Angels, inviting them to her concerts and even singing at one of their parties before finally becoming disillusioned. She sabotaged or undermined every potentially stable relationship with lovers, friends, and relatives because of her drug and alcohol use, her sexual promiscuity and her extreme, chaotic lifestyle. At the same time many of her friends and colleagues seemed quite tolerant of her behavior, as though they sensed her to be a tormented, still innocent girl who was more deserving of empathy than condemnation.

This complicated personality, with all its contradictions and inner agonies, proved to be a powerhouse of energy who became a new, original song stylist and interpreter of folk, blues, jazz and country music. As we previously noted, she pulled her audiences to her with a compelling emotional intensity. Sometimes, especially in her last year or two, she openly encouraged her concert audiences to sing, dance and make love. Her audiences loved her and expected her to be irreverent. She talked directly to them, urging them to "get it on" between and even during songs about sex and life. For a sense of how she affected her audiences, see the captivating pair of photographs by Bill Higgins in the Myra Friedman book, capturing someone from the audience reaching up onstage to touch Janis' hand.

Janis would take a swing at anyone who insulted her or exhibited threatening behaviors, and she was punched out herself on occasion. Irony and tragedy are to be found in her life as well as in Morrison's. Each died at a time when the condition with which they struggled was being actively investigated and articulated.

In fact as early as 1967, Otto Kernberg identified patients whose internal psychological structures he labeled "borderline personality organizations." Around the mid-seventies, clinical research on the diagnosis and treatment of these disorders was well under way and yielding impressive results. Kernberg was developing a modification of psychoanalysis called "expressive psychotherapy," and by 1974 clinical communities were progressing rapidly in their capabilities to treat borderline patients. One cannot help but wonder what might have been, for example, had Janis been treated by Dr. Kernberg at Cornell University or Dr. Gunderson at Harvard University, who was also exploring borderline conditions.

Janis is known to have seen a mental health professional on two or three occasions. She asked to be admitted to a psychiatric hospital in 1965, insisting that she felt "crazy." At that time she had been using amphetamines, which would have intensified her inner turmoil, while causing a serious deterioration in her mental functioning. According to Friedman's account, the hospital refused to admit her because she was perceived to be malingering, looking for a place to sleep.

In an earlier episode in Texas, she saw a clinical social worker because she was concerned about her drug use and her emerging need to control herself. Apparently deciding that her level of pathology was significant, the clinician who saw her that day described Janis as "diffused" — one of the symptoms of a disordered personality. He warned her about the attendant costs to her mental health posed by the pressures of performing. However, aside from the caution he urged her to exercise, and lacking any conceptual framework which might permit a more insightful analysis of her condition, he could not offer her an effective treatment.

As we worked to understand Janis we found

ourselves imagining how her fate might have been different had she been accurately evaluated and effectively treated. After researching his life, it is our sense of Jim Morrison that he would have been a more difficult candidate for psychotherapy than Janis. It is simply difficult to imagine him seeking help. He so completely engaged his intellect in the pursuit of the "dark side," so assuredly saw the problems of his life as emanating from outside himself, and was so hostile to convention that he simply would have engaged in verbal warfare with the therapist. Although his lifelong antisocial behavior and hostility are personality traits associated with poor outcome in psychotherapy, we think nevertheless he would have been a challenging and interesting patient.

We believe that the emerging models of borderline conditions that have recently become available to therapists have greatly enhanced their success with such patients. In this chapter we offer an informed look at what several psychotherapeutic sessions with Janis might have been like. Could she have been helped? Or would she have frustrated the process as so many like her have done?

Imagine if you can, the following course of psychotherapy as we have constructed it for Janis, and later Jim, based on our sense of them from what others have written and on a modern clinical understanding of the various borderline conditions. Using my own experiences with these kinds of patients, I (GAF) present portions of five different sessions with Janis, a first, eleventh, twelfth, twentieth and twenty-eighth, to illustrate how the process might have evolved with her. I use my own theoretical framework and clinical style, attempting to portray her in a manner consistent with her recorded dialogue, individual idiosyncrasies and the records of her life experiences.

Janis is sent by her friends and associates who are worried about her drug and alcohol abuse, fluctuating emotional states, and agitated state of mind. She has agreed to see a clinician because she too is now concerned about her drug abuse. She has also become more depressed of late and as always, is very lonely.

Session 1.

It is late September of 1970, one week after twenty-seven year old Jimi Hendrix choked to death under circumstances involving drug use (Janis died two weeks later at age 27. Jim Morrison nine months later, also at age 27). She is dressed in her uniquely Janis clothes designed by Linda Gravenites (Friedman 1973, 87-88), including love beads, bracelets, boa ala Bessie Smith, and sandals. She is overweight, has acne on her face, and looks exhausted. There is something childlike about her despite her well known use of rough language and the dramatic way she presents herself.

GAF: Please come in.
(We shake hands. Her hand feels firm but tense; not unusual for a first visit to a therapist. I note her hip clothes and her attempt to appear casual and easy. Further, not being a rock fan at that time, I have no knowledge of Janis Joplin and Jim Morrison. However, we can assume she would have expected me to have been aware of her popularity and her music. Nervously she looks around, smiling, and giggling slightly.

*She sits down and looks amusingly at
my office arrangement. I explain briefly
how the therapy process works. Then
we begin.)*
Why do you think you need to see
me?

Janis: Well I'm not sure doc, my friends
think I need some help. *(A brief
sample of her famous cackle laugh, then
sadly)* And I feel really down a lot.
*(Another pause, then a quick change of
mood.)* By the way doc, who does
your decorating?

GAF: How do you mean? *(With raised
eyebrows.)*

Janis: Well, it's a bit dull in here. You
could use a lot more color and
some curtains to start with.

GAF: Really?
*(Janis was widely known to be
gregarious, impulsive, and dramatic,
features consistent with a 'hysterical'
type of personality someone who, for
example, becomes "familiar" with
strangers quickly.)*

Janis: Yeah, you need something to
make it real, things here and there,
to . . . like make it alive, man. I
mean, you know, more groovy.
*(Her emotional state changes again and
after a long pause and some more*

*looking around, she is moved back to
the subject at hand by the therapist's
silence.*) I don't know why . . . don't
know why I do some of the things I
do. I'm trying to have a good time
. . .It's just that I, you know . . feel .
. . I don't know . . . really bad most
of the time. (*Janis stares out the
window, her head moving slowly,
despairingly from side to side. The skin
on her face seems loose and sagging.
Her body lies sprawled in the chair as if
thrown there like a discarded coat*).

GAF: Uh huh.

Janis: You know, like I've got all these
people around, friends, chicks,
and cats . . . and they're cool, but
they're never really there when
you need them. Especially the
cats. They're all users. I get it on a
lot but it doesn't last. (*More "cool"
jargon followed by another moment of
sadness, then another shift.*) So, do
you like rock, blues, jazz, or what?

GAF: Why do you ask?

Janis: Oh just curious. (*She then recites a
litany of complaints about uptight and
boring people, society, prejudices, cats,
chicks and the general unfairness of
life. She is very animated and intense,
very articulate and clearly well read.
Yet at the same time, in her tone and*

choice of words, she has somehow managed to let me see her unrelenting anxiety_and agitation. Janis is apt to act overtly and become verbal, physical, or emotional rather than simply withdraw in order to contain her demons.)
Well, what do you think?

GAF: Mmm. Why don't we just continue?

Janis: Yeah, but can you help me?

GAF: I don't know yet. Tell me more about yourself.

Janis: Yeah okay. I . . . it's hard man . . . I mean things seem, sometimes I feel like I can't . . . can't *(pensive, silent, then resumes)* I think sometimes it's just too much. Maybe Jimi had it right.

GAF: Jimi?

Janis: Yeah, Jimi Hendrix. They say he choked to death last week. At least he went out famous. We made it for a while last year, he was right on, man. I'm getting fed up too . . . just tired of all the bullshit. And everybody thinks I use too much.

GAF: Uh huh. Do you?

Janis: I don't know. I can handle it. But I need it, man. I need it . . . *(Again a desperate look, an imperceptible shudder from this tormented human being.)*

GAF: What do you use?

Janis: Heroin mostly. And downers.

GAF: Other drugs?

Janis: I tried speed but its not for me. And I don't do acid or grass anymore either.

GAF: How come?

Janis: I feel terrible on uppers, like weird and nervous. And grass makes me think too much. I saw a social worker in Texas once when I was trying to shake the uppers. He was helpful, but I still . . . I don't know.

GAF: Uh huh. How about alcohol?

Janis: Yeah . . . alcohol, too. It helps.

GAF: Helps?

Janis: You know, it just helps.

GAF: Helps what?

Janis: I don't know, it just helps. Jesus! *(After a short silence)* Well? *(Looking worried now)* Aren't you gonna say something? What do you want me to say? I just need it. I just need it. All I want is a little peace. . . *(Her words become almost inaudible as she pensively looks out of the window. Janis slumps back, frowns at me and throws her boa on the floor. Even in this moment of reflection she seems to be sitting too still, like a coiled spring on the verge of expansion.)* . . . just a little fucking peace.

GAF: Peace?

Janis: Yeah, a little peace. (*Again frowning and impatient.*)

GAF: Peace from what?

Janis: I don't know, I'm always . . . I don't know. I don't know, it just never stops. I'm on edge all the time.

GAF: What never stops?

Janis: The bullshit, the goddamn bullshit. I mean like it's hard man, it's just hard. Never quiet, never peaceful. Always, you know . . . like uneasy. It used to be more fun sometimes, but now it's just. . . I don't know, man . . . it's all fucked up. Nothing feels good anymore. I don't know, I think I'm going crazy. Can't get to feeling really groovy, not ever. I'm just . . . always uneasy. And just don't lecture me about drugs, I know what I'm doing and I'm careful.

GAF: Uneasy?

Janis: Yeah, uneasy. It's always the same no matter what. I'm really down most of the time. *(long silence)* It's hopeless. I don't know . . .

GAF: *Silence*

Janis: *(stares)* Yeah. It's like hopeless, man, just hopeless, and . . . lonely, like nothing. . . like something's missing. Yeah, like I'm bored, really bored, and, oh Fuck. So is it hopeless? *(nervous laugh)*. What can I do about it? *(Now, Janis is trying to get away from her hopeless mood. She brightens up, recovers from the slumped position, picks up her boa and resumes eye contact with me.)*

GAF: Well, we'll try and find out.

Janis: Okay. What else do you want to know?

GAF: What else would you like to tell me?

Janis: Are you ever going to answer a question? Well let's see, I was born dirt poor in a small, cold, shack. *(smiles jokingly, now, with her eyes wide open while she leans forward in the seat.)* Okay, I'm from Port Arthur, Texas. I have one sister and one brother. My father is a great guy, a secret intellectual. My mother is a lot of things, musical, smart, a great teacher.

GAF: Uh huh.

Janis: I've got a new album out. Working on a groovy new one, "Buried Alive in the Blues." *(There's a long silence. Of course this is an ironic choice of titles considering her emotional state.)* Do you have many VIP patients?

GAF: What makes you ask? *(Considering Janis' risk for suicide, I wonder about her VIP question and whether it is connected with her previous comment about Jimi Hendrix.)*

Janis: Oh, no reason, just curious.

GAF: You mentioned Jimi Hendrix?

Janis: Yeah. He was cool man. He did some great things and then checked out at his peak. That's how he'll be remembered.

GAF: Is that how you're feeling?

Janis: Naw, just thinking about it. Besides, Jimi stole the show for this year. But I can't stand much more of this shit. I just can't stand it. I mean, everything feels like shit . . . can't ever just . . . *(She begins to look depressed and becomes agitated. After a brief silence, she looks up and, with the wave of her hand, tries to shake off the question but quickly begins to look depressed and becomes mildly agitated.)* So what now? What do I do now?

GAF: You're feeling like shit now?

Janis: Yeah, so what? You fucking shrinks are all alike, never answer a question straight. *(Now becoming more irritated, rapidly twiddling her fingers).*

GAF: Is this what you mean by being on edge? *(Together with the sudden shifts in emotion, her quickness to anger and to becoming incensed with me – a stranger, afterall, whose help she is seeking.–I now suspect the presence of serious pathology.)*

Janis: *(Just looks at me, now calmly, as if my observation relieved some of the tension).* Yeah . . . I guess so . . . yeah. *(Mood shifts and she smiles wanly.)*

Janis: *(Looking out window, slowly becoming sad again and wistful. After a long while).* So what's the matter with me anyway?

GAF: How do you mean?

Janis: You've had other patients like me?

GAF: Yes, but what is it like for you?

Janis: Uh . . . I don't know, never thought about it before. *(Twirling her bracelets around and around.)*

GAF: Uh huh.

Janis: Guess it's the way I've always been. Even when I'm having a blast, it's like . . . always there.

GAF: Even when you're having a blast?

Janis: Yeah, all the time. It never fucking stops. I get that way even on stage sometimes when things slow down. It's strange. That I never thought much about it before. It's really fucking awful. *(Another long pause, and her face takes on a look of newfound puzzlement, with raised eyebrows and wrinkled forehead.)*

Maybe Jimi felt like this, too.

GAF: *(I try to help Janis clarify her behavior patterns.)* Are you aware of wanting to drink when you're having those awful feelings? Or take drugs?

Janis: Yeah, like after a show I look for a party cause I can't stand to just go home and do nothing. It's too . . . lonely . . . or empty . . . or something. So I wanna have a good time, find a cat I can ball, you know, have a blast. But you're right, I always feel kinda . . . it's a bummer man, a real bummer.

GAF: Uh huh.

Janis: You know, the same thing happens with drugs. It's like . . . the same thing man, it's all the same fucking thing. It's really bad . . . feeling so lonely, I mean. All the time, man, all the time and . . . oh, man! *(She stares out window, tears well up)*

GAF: *(Janis is working well on her own. Comments from me are unnecessary at this point as they might interfere with her mood and associations. So I acknowledge her feelings with a neutral response which just restates her words and then I remain silent)* Mmmm.

You mean you party, have sex,
and do drugs when you're feeling
like shit or on edge?

Janis: Yeah, that's right. All I want is
some peace from this . . . this
fucking whatever it is! Jesus
Christ! . . . I'm so tired, so tired.
(Another long silence) I can't believe
this.

GAF: Believe what?

Janis: That this is happening, like I'm all
fucked up. Why do I always feel
so bad? Like I don't belong
anywhere. If it doesn't get better
than this then the hell with it. It's
just too lonely all the time, no
matter what I do. *(Interestingly two
of her songs are A Woman Left Lonely
and All is Loneliness.)* And what am
I doing here with a shrink, a
goddamn shrink, like I'm a fucking
schizo? I don't need this shit. *(Janis
stares angrily at the floor and once
again discards the boa. She slowly
looks up at me as if expecting an
answer to her comments.)*

GAF: Silence

Janis: How come you just sit there?
Don't you have anything to say?
What do you think? Jesus. I'm
here trying to get my fucking head

together and you're just sitting
there. *(Eyebrows arching angrily and
on the edge of the seat leaning toward
me.)*

GAF: If you remember, we discussed at
the beginning of the session how
this therapy works. I'll be
listening to you carefully and
trying to understand what you are
telling me. I'll offer you my
thoughts when I think they might
be helpful to you.

Janis: Yeah, *(Janis caves in the face of this
mild reminder)* sorry. I remember.
Okay. It's really strange, though.
I've always lived my life full tilt . .
like the name of my band. Some
artists separate their private from
their professional lives, but I never
have. I go all out, no limits. Some
of my friends think I'll try
anything. I'm out for fun and I've
done it all and do it all. So why
am I so very miserable most of the
time? It's awful, just awful. I've
had a very successful year on
stage, I have a funky house,
clothes, I must've balled fifty cats,
(typical Janis Joplin bravado) had tons
of booze and drugs, and I still feel
like shit all the time, this boredom,
this emptiness. Why's this
happening to me, huh doc?

GAF: Maybe we can figure it out together.

Janis: Yeah . . . Okay. It's just that I get so lonely. And I'm driven. I don't know why I do things.

GAF: Do things?

Janis: Yeah, I get groovin and anything goes. People tell me I have a filthy mouth and no sense of moderation. I guess I'm an extremist. *(Silence)* I meet all kinds of people in my work, all the rock artists and show business types. *(Stares off vaguely)* You really think we can do something about this? Really? *(Without waiting for response, Janis settles down and moves on to another subject.)* So, do you like rock, or jazz, or blues? I hope you're not too boring.

GAF: How do you mean?

Janis: Well, if we're going to work together . . . I was just curious.

This first session went very well. Janis was more emotionally temperate than she would be in subsequent sessions. She learned for the first time to try to comprehend her inner state of feeling and that there might be a way of understanding it. And she seemed to have become somewhat comfortable with me, joking and poking fun, and at the end, deciding to continue. Unlike the therapists of the sixties, I possess a clinical framework for conceptualizing and treating her condition, a significant advantage. After only one session, I begin to suspect that her "boredom" and "uneasiness" and "loneliness" are common feelings expressed by those experiencing the dead zone. But further assessment is needed.

Sessions 2 through 9

Through more history taking, I expand on the material gathered in the first session, attempting to clarify Janis' experiences of emptiness and impulsivity. She takes the therapist to task again for his boring taste in decor while she repeatedly complains about her bad luck with men, providing a detailed description of her latest relationship with Seth Morgan. She continues to express the hope for a quick, magical cure for her feelings of despair, leaving the session hopeful but anxious. We have agreed to meet three times each week.

Indirectly seeking again to learn whether I have heard of her, she talks about the rock scene she knows so well and her latest performance. Together we examine her continual use of drugs and alcohol.

Session 10.

Janis doesn't show, but by now I am becoming more certain that she is suffering from a borderline syndrome.

Session 11.

Janis arrives dressed more conservatively than in the first few sessions, her hair styled in a more restrained fashion, her mood upbeat. Appreciative of my work with her, she seems to be genuinely interested in continuing her therapy. She makes, however, no mention of missing the previously scheduled hour.

Janis: (*Immediately on entering*) Feeling good today, Doc. But you were right last session about me and smack. I gotta stop. Went and used minutes after I left your office. Don't even know why. Just wanted some. (*Janis is puzzled, perhaps for the first time, consciously reflecting on her drug abuse. We had previously discussed her loneliness, how she seemed either to be attracted to unstable men or to drive stable men away. We had then tied her actions to her need for drugs and she seemed to "get it," although it's uncertain just what she "got." She looks brighter than last time and her eyes flash playfulness and exuberance as she slides into the leather recliner, putting her legs over one arm and pulling the lever to open the leg rest.*)

GAF: Right after you left my office? Do you remember how you were feeling?

Janis: Well, I was headed for a recording session. Remember, I told you about it?   It's going to be FAN-tastic. And I told you before that my last one is doing great. *(Janis is still searching for ways to find out what I might think of her work.)* And I needed something. I know everyone is down on me for using. And Uncle Albert *(Albert Grossman, her manager)* isn't cool about it either. He gets like, all crazy when he thinks his stars are using. *(Notice how she lets me know about her star status. Most borderline patients have strong narcissistic tendencies.)*

GAF: You needed something?

Janis: Yeah, you know, like just needed to, uh, you know, just uh . . . so what? Jesus! You're always at it. I can't stand it. You've always got to question everything. Can't you just take it for what it is? *(Janis is quite irritated with me. She would like to go on narrating her story and having my full attention. When I raise questions she is reminded of why she is there, and it spoils her fantasies of impressing me.)* Haven't you ever read Ferlinghetti or Kerouac or anything but those goddamn textbooks? Does everything have to be Freudian? I told you that I can handle it. I just wanted to let you know that you were right about me using after our sessions. Can't you just give me a little credit for something? What is it with you?

GAF: Well, you say you needed something right after you left my office, and I wondered about how you were feeling then. I wondered if it's perhaps hard for you to leave each time?

Janis: *(A long silence)* Yeah, so what? *(Becoming very quiet now and almost inaudible.)* Yeah, I do feel like that, uh . . . I don't want to go, like I want to stay longer. *(Once again Janis seems to shrink in size and appears lost in the chair. I find it hard to avoid thinking of her as a sad and scared little girl.)*

GAF: So when you do walk out the door, what are you feeling?

Janis: Uh . . . I guess it's uh, it's just . . . it's like shit, man, like shit! Fucking lousy, empty. . . . *(Janis begins to get in touch with the feeling.)*

GAF: Empty, is that the feeling we've been talking about?

Janis: Yeah, I guess so, I guess so, it's really hard to describe.

GAF: So when you're here you feel better and when you leave here you feel alone and empty?

Janis: Yeah. I can't stand it, it's like a goddamn nightmare and you're the only one who can stop it, here in your office. And there I am, leaving. Everything ends until the next session. So I go looking for friends and some smack and try to keep going till the next session. Like there's nothing else but here. Everything seems so goddamn unimportant, so unreal. I just want to get by until I'm back here. Can't you do something? What is this, why am I like this? Why me? Jesus! (*Tears well up again and it's easy to see that she's angry. She frowns and become agitated.*)

GAF: So you need drugs to take away the uneasy feelings . . except that they take away all your feelings?

Janis: Right on. And you, you're hard, man. You stick to the time like you don't care. (*Janis is now escalating emotionally and mocks me.*) We have to stop now, we have to stop now. . . like your time is so fucking important. Well my time is, too, man. I have a tight schedule just as important as your is, you think you're so goddamn cool. So smart, like you know it all. Well, fuck you man, just fuck off with all your questions. *(Now Janis is in a full blown outburst, staring at me, the expression on her face filled with rage.)* I don't need this, fuck this, what do you want from me anyway? Asshole! Fuck you! Fuck you!

GAF: You'd prefer it if I didn't follow the rules with you, made an exception? *(I remain unruffled, silently communicating to her that I can withstand her anger, and that I will resolutely seek to determine what it all means.)*

Janis: *(Screaming now)* I don't care what the fuck you do. You're just in this for the money like everybody else. *(After standing up and pacing around the room she hurls another "fuck you" and "fucking asshole", then leaves, slamming the door and cursing as she charges down the corridor.)*

This is a good example of the complexity of working with this kind of patient. Janis clearly was experiencing the intense and dreadful feeling of abandonment, the central feeling of the dead zone, each time our sessions ended.

It is typical for borderline personalities to form quick, intense attachments to people and become very dependent and demanding. It is also common for many of them to have unpredictable outbursts for no apparent reason (because of what is going on internally). She became enraged when I maintained the boundaries of the therapy by staying on schedule because she felt entitled to special treatment, and because she felt her ever present emptiness and despair upon separating from the therapist. Yet any violation of the strict boundaries of therapy would make her worse.

Her reaction was to seek escape, in this case by drug use. When I attempted to connect the feelings of abandonment with her use of drugs, she "got it" and felt understood for a moment, and thus more connected to me. But this only made leaving at the end of the hour that much more dreadful, and she exploded in rage. Considering that this is the first time Janis has been given any hope of bringing her sense of inner despair under control, one is reminded of the axiom some have applied to the treatment of borderline patients: "no good deed will go unpunished."

Session 12.

Janis arrives on time, calm and matter of fact. Her weight is up and her eyes are ringed and bloodshot. She raises the incident of the previous hour and her stormy exit.

Janis: So what's up? I suppose you want to talk about last time. You always want to *understaaand* everything. Maybe some things are just what they are. Maybe this is just intellectual masturbation. Maybe none of this means anything. *(Janis's sarcasm betrays the anger still there.)*

GAF: It would help if we could sort out what happened last time.

Janis: I don't know, I just felt pissed off. *(Drawn and demoralized, she lowers her head, gazing only at the floor. She has clearly been having a hard time.)*

GAF: You seemed all right until we began talking about how dreadful you feel at the end of each session. Could it be that you've been angry about always having to leave, about always feeling that way, and finally let go of the feeling?

Janis: I guess I do get pissed off after I leave here, even if I liked what we talked about. *(Janis leans forward, her elbows on her knees, chin cupped in palm of her hand, and eyes looking up with eyebrows raised. She is sad, puzzled and perhaps a little embarrassed.)*

GAF: Perhaps that's why you missed the session before last? *(I'm certain of what happened now and it will help Janis to know that I know.)*

Janis: What do you mean?

GAF: Maybe you stayed away to protect me from your wrath, from your anger at having to leave? *(I say this in a bit of a whisper for effect.)*

Janis: Goddamn! *(Smiling sheepishly)* You know about that. How do you know about that? I was so fucking pissed, I could've punched your face in. So I didn't come.

GAF: You were being considerate. You wanted to be sure you wouldn't injure me.

Janis: Yeah *(still smiling)* daddy, that's right. *Janis softens, sits back in the chair and moves on. The change in her mood is striking. She is no longer appears grim and fatigued. Instead a smile breaks out, and her tone is upbeat and playful.)* So, what shall we talk about today? Want to hear about my sex life? *(Janis is teasing me and bragging at the same time.)*

GAF: Silence. *(A patient like Janis will fill our sessions with grist for the mill, material for the therapeutic process. All I have to do is wait.)*

Janis: Well? *(Teasing)* What's the matter, doc, don't you like sex? I've balled all kinds of cats man, and chicks, too. Can't seem to get enough. I thought you were Freudian? It's all about sex isn't it? I mean, everybody's lookin to get laid. I'm just very good at it. But I never get enough. Always lookin'. Are you gettin enough, doc? Are you like me—never enough? (*Janis thinks she's on safer ground with sex, and knows her way around 'the scene'.*)

GAF: Enough?

Janis: Yeah, enough. I get laid all the time, and I'm always looking for new . . . talent. And I still want more action. It doesn't last long after so I have to keep lookin'.

GAF: Mmm. Well, you make it sound like you have a voracious sexual appetite. But how is it that you're still wanting if you're getting laid all the time? (*I'm asking her to confront a contradiction here—she gets lots of sex but it doesn't last her very long. It appears that she is driven by the prospect of obtaining sexual gratification while she freely concedes that she is insatiable. I give no consideration to the idea that she is just a "very sexual person" as some of my patients have insisted. It seems clear enough from her accounts that sex is being used here like so many other things—food, alcohol, work, physicality to name a few—as a means of escaping inner confusion or conflict.*)

Janis: I don't know, I'm just after it all the time. What's the difference? Are you going to tell me that sex is bad? Am I supposed to be virginal and a good little girl? Come on, doc, are you really that straight? I want it all the time and that's just the way it is. Take love where you find it. It may not be here tomorrow. *(These lines, of course are drawn from the music she wrote.)*

GAF: Is that the same reason you're after drugs and alcohol?

Janis: I guess so. *(Puzzled once again, Janis looks at me wondering where I'm headed with this line of questions.)*

GAF: Maybe there's more to it.

Janis: What do you mean? Sex is sex and I'm not repressed about it. The country is so uptight about sex, but I'm not buying into that crap. I'm not buying into the white house with the picket fence and all the girls are virgins crap. It's phony and hypocritical, and I have to tell it like it is. *(Reacting self-righteously)* So what do you mean there's more to it? *(Acting as if she were annoyed once again)*

GAF: There's sex and there's driven sex.

You make it sound as though you're driven.

Janis: Well, a little maybe, I guess so. So what? It's all the same anyway man, all the same shit. How else do you expect it to be? What else is there? It's that or be lonely all the fucking time. *(Long silence. She may be feeling that I'm raining on her parade again, taking away self-perspectives that were of some comfort to her.)*

GAF: What about love, sharing experiences, affection, friendship, feeling connected? What you describe as sex doesn't seem to have much connectedness. Only the physical.

Janis: Well, yeah, maybe. *(Wistfully)* But I did connect with a few guys and some other people.

GAF: If I recall our discussions, you always pick troublesome men or behave so as to cause problems for any serious, straight relationship. Do I have that right? *(Janis lets me proceed. She is curious about where I'm going.)*

Janis: Yeah, I guess so. I always seem to be too much—too much my own person and they can't handle that.

Besides, the straight ones are usually boring. *(The problem she is describing expressed in clinical terms is that, for Janis, relationships without conflict are not intense enough to suppress the feelings from the dead zone. What is significant here is Janis's tendency to dismiss her own behaviors as having anything to do with her problems. This is a good example of her narcissistic side, again common in borderline patients).*

GAF: Could it be that you're driven about sex for the same reasons that you are driven to use drugs and alcohol?

Janis: You mean the emptiness, the dead feeling?

GAF: Yes. You said it never stops.

Janis: *(A long pause, after which she slowly shakes her head from side to side, then quietly)* Oh man . . . sometimes I don't care who it is, only that they're there and ready. It's the loneliness, I can't stand the loneliness. It's too hard and I get bored too and . . . uh . . . I get unbearably tense, yeah! *(Another long silence)* So that's it, isn't it? Like booze and drugs, I use sex to deal with it—the fucking emptiness? You're right, I dread it,

88

I'll do anything. Anything. Anything. *(Looking very upset now.)* I mean. . . doc, like sometimes I don't even feel alive, feel real. Like there's no me, no nothing! Like something's missing.

GAF: Uh huh. Those feelings are partly responsible for your tensions and for your need to behave in extremes. It seems that it takes intense stimulation and excitement to help block those feelings.

Janis: Sex and drugs.

GAF: Yes. *(It will take awhile and many reminders before Janis will be able to remember this sex and drugs connection in her daily life. Only then will we be able to find ways to help.)*

Janis: *(Now slumped in the chair, Janis is both pensive and sad. She looks quite small and fragile. The tough, wisecracking, modern day Bessie Smith of earlier sessions is temporarily subdued. Clarifying once again the relationship between her behavior and feelings of emptiness is having some affect for the moment.)* So what can I do? Am I hopeless?

GAF: We have to explore this together to see what we can do.

Janis: Okay. Let's do it. I can't stand the thought that it's going to be like this forever. I'd rather be dead. This is worse than dead. Everywhere I go I get down, sooner or later I get down. It's a goddamn bummer. All I want is to get my fucking head together, man, that's all. That's all. I gotta get my head together, gotta feel real.

GAF: Real?

Janis: Real, I don't know what I mean. It's just that I'm never sure I'm there, except maybe on stage . . . oh fuck. I don't know how to explain it, I just don't feel as though there's a me, as though I really exist. *(Janis looks very anxious and desperate.)*

During this session Janis identified and clarified the feelings she associated with the dead zone. She lacked the inner resources needed to soothe herself and to feel "real" and alive. Typical of borderline patients, she seemed unable to hold within herself the internalized images (representations) of the nurturing caretakers of childhood. This holding environment is a precondition necessary for all of us to regulate our emotional states, especially the experience of loneliness. Helping her to see more of her outrageous behaviors as symptoms of this devastating barrenness of her inner world gives her hope and direction.

Janis' futile efforts to find the internal resources

to soothe herself and feel "real" left her, as always, despondent. Shortly after she began therapy, perhaps by the fifth or sixth session, she found that calling me to check in and hear my voice calmed her panicky feelings somewhat and improved her sense of being real (if I really existed then so did she). On her own she could not manage her crushing emptiness, the terrifying world of the dead zone. Her agonizing need for connectedness could not be gratified, because actual connecting would cause her to feel the threat of losing herself — her very existence — in the other person. On the other hand, her rage and hostility at the expectation of abandonment created an ever-changing, shifting internal state. Life was experienced as polarized: extreme attachments, extreme disappointments, extreme anger, and extreme anxieties. All of these needful feelings and internal demon images were regularly projected onto people involved with her, making stable relationships impossible.

Session 20.

Janis by this time (two months later at three times per week) is struggling with the vicissitudes of the therapeutic process. People will eventually act out their real conflicts, personality style, and tendencies in therapy, and Janis did so more quickly and more intensely than most.

Janis' intense "affect storms" of despair, anxiety, and outrage were difficult to contain in the first few months. She proved to be challenging, obstreperous, seductive, demanding, and infantile, as well as charming, warm, responsive, and entertaining. She struggled heroically to keep her psychic balance. I made every effort to follow her internal state of mind, help her identify the emptiness and disconnectedness behind her pain and bring her some relief. How difficult this was to accomplish, and the patience required to follow the endless twists and turns of her emotional roller coaster, is again illustrated in the next session.

The previous two sessions were relatively calm for Janis as she reviewed her career and her love of singing, performing and the limelight. In addition to shifting emotional states, she alternately gained and lost weight, and the severity of her acne waxed and waned. Her clothing varied too, with her appearing in a lengthy but simple hippie dress in one session, and during another in a heavily beaded, multicolored outfit set off by a feathered boa. These wildly fluctuating, highly ostentatious modes of dressing, along with chaotic behaviors, are symptomatic of the erratic functioning of some borderline personalities. Clinicians often refer to that personality pattern as "stably unstable."

Janis arrived for this session in a cantankerous mood and somewhat disarrayed. She did not mention her phone call to me on the previous evening when she had felt frightened and wretched, and had vaguely threatened "not to put up with it" anymore.

Janis: *(She plops down, impatiently waiting for me to say something. Her arm has a pretty good size bandage on it and she is obviously unsettled as she moves about restlessly in the chair.)* Well. Say something, you're just staring at me.

GAF: I see that you're not in a good mood.

Janis: *(Softens)* Naw, I'm just not in the mood for anything. I'm just tired, tired of people using me. Nobody really gives a damn about me, doc. Nobody really loves me. I'm sick of it. *(In a whiny, pleading voice now).* How come everybody leaves me? Everybody. The only people who love me are people who work for me, and then only 'cause I pay them.

GAF: What's happened since Monday? *(After our last meeting, two days ago, Janis left in an upbeat mood. While not surprised at her quick change in mood, I must try to determine what triggered it).*

Janis: Same old shit. Tried to get it on after a recording session Tuesday. We were out all night with some of the guys and I ended up kicking them out. All they did was drink my stuff and try to rob me blind. Fuckers. Jesus, I couldn't even get laid. They had grass, but I got wasted on booze and fell down the stairs in my own goddamn house. Look at this cut on my arm. I spent half the night in the fucking emergency room waiting for them to sew it up. Jesus. And a lot of my friends are gone — Nancy, Peggy, Kris . . . and Linda's mad at me, she hates drugs. I don't know, I'm just so tired, doc, just so tired.

GAF: Uh huh. So this all happened after the recording session? Is that what you usually do afterward? Party all night?

Janis: Sure, getting it on, man. Have a ball, you know. Jesus, are you straight. But things are getting harder. It's really bad. I'm feeling bad all the time. I can't stand being down all the time I mean . . . fuck, nobody cares. If it keeps up I'm gonna end it, it's just too fucking much. (*Staring angrily at the floor.*)

GAF: Now wait. Help me understand this better. Walk me through the events, beginning with the recording session.

Janis: You know, it was a rehearsal session. We were getting ready for my new album and then had some fun with a few old songs and a few new ones that we're trying out. It was after one a.m. and I was fucking exhausted. But a couple of the guys had their chicks hanging around and decided to get stoned. I can't stand that shit, gets my head all fucked up. Anyway, I invited everybody to my place, everybody. Four of the guys hopped in my car and we headed out. Then we get stopped by a cop who didn't like the looks of my car. *(Janis has a brightly painted psychedelic Porsche.)* The cop spots my bottle, smelled my breath and handed me a ticket. He wouldn't let us move until one of the others got behind the wheel. He started giving me some jive shit about drinking and driving with this sneer on his face. So I jumped up to go after him and whack him with the bottle, but one of the guys pushed me down and sat on me till the cop got to his cruiser. He followed us all the way to my house. But then the party started and we had a blast until one of those obtuse fucking chicks came at me because she thought I was trying to get it on with her man. Big deal. I still don't know why she threw a fit. They had to pull me off her. I kicked her out and went down to get some smack. That's when I tripped on the stairs. I almost broke my neck and ended up in the emergency room with this cut. It took twelve stitches to sew my arm. When I got back everybody who left was stoned out of their mind and the place was trashed. I kicked the whole bunch of them out on their collective asses.

GAF: How did you come to decide to invite everyone to your house?

Janis: What? (*Annoyed and puzzled with wrinkled brow.*)

GAF: I was wondering how, after a long day, and at one a.m., you felt like partying when you were already exhausted?

Janis: *(Mildly irritated)* I don't know. What difference does it make? We were doing it . . . getting it on . . . getting down, man. Sex, booze, drugs with my friends. That's what we do, man, that's making the scene. We would have gone to one of our hangouts, too, if those fuckers hadn't pulled that shit.

GAF: Do you ever just go home after a session?

Janis: No, man. That's when we party. I can't believe you, Jesus. Were you ever young? Don't you like having a good time? Don't you like fucking? Booze? Jeez. What do you do for fun, doc, or don't you like fun? Jeez. (*Janis is upset by my questions. She doesn't feel supported at this moment and turns away from me in the chair.*)

GAF: Then you'll party even if you're exhausted? *(I confront an incongruity: She needs to keep going, looking for excitement even when she's exhausted.)*

Janis: So? What are you getting at? I'm usually wound up after the sessions and after concerts. Could keep going all night. It's hard to stop. Everybody's feeling wasted and looking to get it on. I mean come on man, this is the scene, it's what's happening. Where the action is. How can you even ask that question? Time to go back to the books, doc. Don't you have a place in your philosophy, in your mind, that allows for people getting it on? Jesus!

GAF: Silence

Janis: So? What . . . what are you getting at? What are you getting at anyway? *(Long silence with Janis staring at me.)* The emptiness, the hole, huh?

GAF: Well, is it possible? *(Janis needs to be reminded about the connection between her behavior and the dead zone. We have discussed it many times, yet she still must be directed to it. She acts up, cavorts, and goes on alcoholic binges while partying, and she is impulsive, impatient, and highly reactive to everything because she uses these behaviors to avoid the unbearable experience of her own silence.)*

Janis: Jeez . . . maybe. Everybody's out there, having a ball and I think that . . . maybe I always feel, really . . . apart from them. *(Janis is looking sad now and her "get it on" bravado dissolves as she becomes more reflective about the meaning of her behavior in this regard.)* And I guess I didn't want to go home alone. I hate it. The nights are the worst. That's when I need smack the most . . . to numb out. You don't know, doc, you don't know how much I hate it . . . being alone, as if there's no one there. I can't even feel me there. Like I'm not, not . . . me. Like hollow, just an imaginary being. Maybe I'm a doppleganger, a ghost. Nothing solid, you can see right through me cause I'm not really here. I'm not really anywhere. I just can't stand it anymore. *(crying quietly, hand on her head tilted to one side.)*

GAF: All the excitement of people, drugs, sex, and fighting —

Janis: Yeah . . . because I'm not alive. I'm not even dead. I'm just . . . not anything. *(Shaking her head, she stares at me a while, remembering many earlier sessions in which we had discussed the same problem.)* I keep forgetting, don't I? What do I do . . . what, how can I get rid of it? Can't you tell me what to do?

GAF: It might help if you could keep it in the front of your mind. You might then recognize it when it starts to disrupt you and causes you to look for distractions. You could then say, Oh, there it is. I can't stand this. What can I do to keep it under control?

Janis: *(Looking up)* Yeah, then what? You've said before that it takes heavy action to block it, like scx, drugs —

GAF: If you can recognize it early then you might be able to find new and better ways to contain it. We'll have to be very creative and experimental. And it would help if your life had more structure to it, more predictability— without cramping your freewheeling style too much. But we still need to keep working to understand your self-destructive behaviors, your tendencies to disrupt relationships and so on.

Janis: Yeah, I can be pretty impossible sometimes. But it really, really gets unbearable, doc. I hope you believe me. I'm not just making it up. I really need *(Teary-eyed and forlorn, Janis slumps in the chair looking both hopeful and scared. She begins to see her problem a little more clearly and wants to have hope despite her remaining skepticism. Her clothes have become a bit disheveled and she absentmindedly tries to straighten up.)*

GAF: I believe you. You were probably scared and feeling desperate like this when you called me yesterday, the day after the party, because you were alone with the emptiness.

Janis: Yeah . . . Yeah . . . it was terrible after everyone left. That's why I called. I couldn't stand it, I, uh . . . I hate to admit it, but I felt much better the minute I heard your voice. I felt real again. It sounds stupid but it was like nothing seemed okay, until I knew that you were really there. I even have your cards all over. Like you're the only thing between me and nothing and I'm barely hanging on. It's crazy. What do I do, call you every time I feel bad? I'd be on the phone all day. So, that's why I have people around all the time. I remember . . . we talked about this. *(Here again is yet another episode in her life that reveals the desolateness of her inner world. Not even her own physical existence can give her a sense of reality in the absence of internal "objects" as mentioned earlier.)*

GAF: Yes, you're in need of connecting with me and yet you're angry with me at the same time? *(A revealing contradiction of the borderline condition.)*

Janis: But I don't want you to be so important to me. It makes me angry, and I want to tell you to fuck off. It's scary because . . . because . . . I don't know. Don't want to be . . . to feel so helpless.

GAF: Could it be that you feel overwhelmed by how strong your feelings of need are, or perhaps that your needs and your rage would destroy me? *(Her exchanges with me here essentially describe the need – fear dilemma. Her overwhelming feelings of need are opposed by an equally overwhelming fear that the need will destroy the person or the needed person.)*

Janis: That's right. If you're gone then I'd . . . like, like I'd have no one. It would be . . . I would be totally alone. Jesus. None of my friends make any difference anymore. They're really no help at all. I'd like to stay in your back pocket. I wouldn't be a bother. I'd just be able to see you and feel safe and real. But then I don't want to be like that—so helpless, so weak. It makes me hate everything, myself, you . . . . Jesus! *(Her torment raw and relentless, Janis begins to sob uncontrollably, obviously scared and utterly miserable.)*

GAF: *(Another clarifying observation is useful here, restating the connections between her inner states and her outer behavior).* Maybe if we can understand it more fully, we can be more effective in helping you.

Janis: Yeah. *(Looking up, eyes red, nose running, she uses a facial tissue and calms down.)* I can't see any way out. The loneliness, it's unbearable. Worse than dead.

GAF: Yes. It appears that you're always feeling those dreadful feelings, the black hole. You feel them when you're alone, when you're with people in a not too stimulating situation, when you're done with a stage performance, when a relationship isn't intense enough, when you're too attached to someone, when you leave my office after a session, when anyone leaves you and when it's time to end the day. You feel it all the time and have felt it as far back as you can remember.

Janis: *(Looking up sadly contemplating my summary, she then finishes the description of her behavior, clearly demonstrating a fine intelligence amidst the anarchy of her life.)* And so I do anything to get away from it. Sex, any sex. Drugs, mostly heroin because it numbs me out, and alcohol because it's easier to use almost anywhere and . . going all-out in my performances on stage. Getting the audience all worked up can numb me to my goddamn misery . . . and when everything else fails I can act up or instigate some kind of disturbance to help out. I'm impulsive, and unpredictable, and create all kinds of trouble that turns people off and fucks up the chances of my having a decent relationship with anybody. I guess that's about it isn't it? My whole life is one big fucking diversion, right . . . just a hopeless attempt to escape from myself. Nothing. Nothing! *(Janis is almost screaming here.)*

GAF: It is a sad situation. But you've

never been able to describe and understand it until now.

Janis: Yeah, sure. So now I'll be better informed when I end it. Jesus, it's unbelievable. Maybe this is all a bunch of crap. Maybe I'm just fucked up, maybe it's too late. *(Janis is hoping I'll contradict her maybes. For most patients with the borderline syndrome, expressing ambivalence is typical; it is not yes or no, but yes and no, not love or hate but love and hate, not alternating or in sequence but at the same time. At this point she is feeling better and worse, more hopeful and more hopeless, all at once. Hence the continuous inner tumult.)*

GAF: Despite your doubts, I wonder if you aren't just a little more hopeful than before?

Janis: Uh . . . yeah I suppose. But you're going on vacation in two weeks. What am I going to do? I can't do this alone. When I leave here today it'll be like every other time. I'll be scared and get to feeling hopeless, and by tonight I won't even exist. *(She starts breathing heavily with increased anxiety).* I can feel it right here now. *(Pointing to her stomach).*

GAF: Let's talk about my vacation and make some arrangements. First, we will have one of my colleagues see you while I'm away. Second, if it becomes necessary, I can be reached on the phone. Third, you should think about setting up a schedule of events for this time — you know, specific dates and times for whatever appropriate activities you choose, like visiting with friends, reading, taking in a play or concert, volunteer work in town. This will bring some needed predictability into your life and reduce your anxiety. Fourth, if you like, we can make a mild tranquilizer available for stressful moments, and something else to help you sleep. Okay?

Janis: *(A little relieved but still apprehensive.)* Yeah . . . that feels a little better. (*She still looks worried and is obviously thinking about my vacation and it's effect on her.*)

GAF: And if you need something to keep the feeling of realness and of being connected, you could try keeping a daily journal of your thoughts and feelings.

Janis: Yeah? I like that, I could do that. Yeah. (*Now Janis is having a moment of hope as she thinks maybe things will work out.*) Thanks Doc.

GAF: Okay.

Janis: See you Friday. (*Lingers, then reluctantly leaves.*)

Janis will have trouble while I'm on vacation. Her experience of my absence will result in irrational, intense feelings of abandonment and rage. She will make several suicidal gestures. On my return, she will act out in various ways, including missing the first session.

Session 28.

Janis misses our first scheduled session after I return from vacation. The next day she leaves word with my answering service that she will make the next session. The next session she enters without comment, but her face tells the story.

She is somber and aloof, her clothes are more colorful and psychedelic than ever, and she has gained some weight. After a period of time when it becomes clear that Janis is maintaining an angry silence, I offer a greeting. Therapy with this kind of patient requires constant attention to the tendency to distort reality, act impulsively, and promote further chaos in her life. Thus the patient will be helped by drawing her attention to the nature of the therapeutic process and to our agreement about her responsibility to collaborate with the therapist.

GAF: Good afternoon.

Janis: (Silence)

GAF: *(After a few more minutes)* You weren't able to keep your scheduled session on Monday.

Janis: Man. What do you think? Things happened. I've gained ten pounds. I've been using heavy and I get drunk every goddamn night. I needed something to get through. Man, you don't know what it's like. I drank and shot up and balled my brains out. I didn't think I'd see you anymore. It still feels that way, even though I see you there. Like . . . it's just that . . . I felt so hopeless. I was ready to cash it in Sunday night. I ended up in the emergency room—booze and smack. One of the guys in the band found me. The doctor at the hospital said I almost died. It's so confusing and I'm so tired . . . so tired. And I know you have a right to take a vacation, and I knew you were coming back, but it still felt like you were gone for good. *(Janis is agitated and angry and scared.)*

GAF: And that made you angry at me. So you didn't come and didn't call.

Janis: Are you serious? I was in the goddamn emergency room. What do you expect? I know it doesn't make sense . . . you were gone and I said to myself, fuck him. He's like all the rest, never coming through, never there when you need them, always promising but never ready to deliver. But I called Tuesday anyway, so what's the big deal?

GAF: Well, you didn't call on Sunday. *(I persist here in describing the facts about her self-destructive behavior without any intention of determining the reasons for it at this time. The point is to make clear that regardless of why she took the actions she did, we cannot work on them if she doesn't come. The message is that she is has a major responsibility for how well her therapy works. As with most patients of this type that I have encountered, Janis is very impulsive, so the structure and requisite psychotherapy are used to provide some containment of her actions so that the therapy can proceed.)*

Janis: But I almost died. How could I call? Jeez!

GAF: I'm referring to the time before you made the decision to take the drugs and alcohol. You know what happens to you when you take drugs. But you didn't follow the agreement made at the beginning of our work together. You were supposed to call me and let me know that you were going to get high, and therefore you weren't coming on Monday.

Janis: Jeez, you expected me to call and tell you that I was planning to overdose? Are you crazy? Why the fuck would I do that? *(Expressing disbelief, she can't imagine how I arrived at my position.)*

GAF: Well, let's review our agreement about the requirements for your work here. It is necessary for the treatment process that you assume responsibility for your life and actions. This form of treatment *(psychoanalytic psychotherapy)* can only work if we meet regularly, and you can't do that if you take actions of any kind that prevent it. So we have to agree on the basic preconditions necessary for this form of therapy. *(I am not expecting Janis to give up her suicidal, self-destructive behavior — that wouldn't work. I am trying to be clear that for her treatment to be successful, she must show up so that her actions can be examined and understood.)*

Janis: Okay, okay. Jeez!

GAF: Well, let's see what we do know. You are prone to impulsive actions and some of these include suicidal behaviors that we cannot dismiss as empty or accidental. We must consider you at great risk. Thus, I expect as one of the preconditions for therapy that whenever you are feeling at risk, no matter what the cause, you go directly to a hospital. *(Here Janis is being apprised that I cannot collude with her wish to be treated in a magical way and be saved by an omnipotent therapist.)*

Janis: So. I went to a hospital.

GAF: Yes, but that was after you overdosed. What I'm saying is this: if you're feeling suicidal and feel unable to control it, then you must go to a hospital. If you feel suicidal and yet still in control, then come to our next session and we'll talk about it.

Janis: What if I've already taken stuff?

GAF: The idea is to do something while you're still conscious and able. If you lose control and act suicidal but are still conscious, then you must call 911 or family or police and go to the hospital. There you'll be evaluated as to the need for further hospitalization, just as the ER doctors did on Sunday.

Janis: Well, why can't you evaluate me then?

GAF: Because once you're out of control, someone else needs to do that. In outpatient therapy my job is to help you toward understanding your problems. If I become involved with managing all of the legal and administrative issues that go along with suicide attempts, I can't fulfill my responsibilities as your outpatient therapist.

Janis: *(After mulling over my comments)* Well, I guess you're the expert. What do we do now? *(Here Janis is feeling helped by the clarity and firmness of my response. She feels more protected from her own actions because my expectations provide her with some structure sorely needed to help contain her own self-destructive impulses.)*

GAF: I had other thoughts about your actions while I was away.

Janis: Yeah? What?

GAF: You could have called but didn't. Dr. Brau was available, but you didn't choose to call her. What can we make of it—of your reluctance to call for help when you felt so bad?

Janis: *(Wrinkles nose and looks away)* I don't know . . . maybe I just didn't think of it.

GAF: Is that the case? Or maybe you were unwilling to call?

Janis: Yeah, that too. I don't feel good about being so needy. I just I hate how pathetic I am. I told you before, I can't even get through a fucking day without calling your office just to listen to your voice on a machine. It's pathetic. Do you know have any idea how humiliating that is? At first I was okay, but then ugh. Even that didn't work. I tried things—like working 20 hours a day. I even went to the goddamn movies for chrissakes. But nothing works. I hate calling, I hate it. I feel so stupid, and I don't even get to talk to you, just the fucking machine. *(Janis sinks deeper into the chair as if needing to be enveloped by it. Long silence.)* Jeez! I gotta have things, people around. Can't you understand, it's like . . . I have people around all day until I go home. If there's no one home or hanging out, I'm . . . it's, I don't know, unbearable! I really, really feel . . . uh, like nothing, like I'm not there, not alive. I need my friends around all the time. You think my life is too hectic, you think partying when I'm exhausted is strange. (*In a louder and more pleading voice.*) Well without them there's nothing! Without you being there, nothing exists! If you're not looking at me or talking to me in person, you don't exist, I don't exist. Can't you understand, can't anybody understand? (*Janis is sobbing uncontrollably. When alone, she cannot have an internal dialogue with the therapist or have a sense of connection or relationship with the therapist because she cannot hold onto any inner "representation" or image of the therapist without the therapist's actual presence. Here is the dilemma and the terror of "object inconstancy", and to some, the true meaning of hell — no internal objects to immunize against the experience of "nothingness."*)

GAF: Silence. (*I let Janis become more consciously aware of the dead zone and its influence on her behavior. My silent attention offers her soothing, nonintrusive company.*)

Janis: (*Janis calms down after a while, but then hopelessness descends.*) I can't do this. I can't do this anymore.

I'm so tired, just tired. What do you want. . .what do you expect me to do? I never feel any different. Do you have any idea how it really is? I always feel like this and . . . I'm always thinking about . . . (*Silence*)

GAF: Suicide. You always have thoughts of suicide?

Janis: Yes. You know, huh? (*Silence*)

GAF: Yes. I know that no matter how well you appear to be, you are never far from feeling the nothingness and the impulse to self-destruct. But we have an agreement, right?

Janis: (*Relieved to learn that I know of her vulnerability.*) Yeah, I know. But it's always there. I always feel deserted. Everybody leaves. Linda's in England. Seth left, Kris left, David left. You left. Where the fuck is everybody going? (*It is Janis's "internal objects" that are leaving. She feels as if she is virtually alone in the universe unless the significant people in her life are readily accessible so she can renew her experience of them.*)

GAF: You can't take your experience of them with you, sort of hold on to

them in your mind?   Feel them
there in your mind?

Janis: You mean, like see them?   Yeah,
man.   But they're not, uh . . . like
anything, not real.   Kinda like
ghosts.

GAF: So your experiences with them
don't last long after you've been
with them?   You have no good
feeling thinking of them?

Janis: Of course not, how can I?   They
aren't real.   I'm not even sure
they're there.   They're like . . . like
. . . I don't know.   It's just, I leave
here and I get along for about a
day or two, then what am I
supposed to do? Camp on your
doorstep?   *(Brief silence.)* What do
you want from me?   I can't do
this — it's too hard.   Do you . . . can
you like, have people in your
mind?   You can do that?   *(Janis
derives   no   benefit   from   any
representations of people that may be in
her mind.   There is no feeling, no
emotional   connection   to   those
representations.   Unlike most of us who
do have feelings and some sense of
attachment to these internal images,
Janis has none.   The images are lifeless.
They cannot soothe.   They leave her in
a dead zone.   This is a kind of object
inconstancy   called   "object*

115

impermanence" where the representation is present without the feelings that are normally associated with them. The result is the experience of lifelessness that Janis is describing.)

GAF: Most people can.

Janis: Jeez. *(Often people in the dead zone do not understand that others do not have the same existential experience as they do.)*

GAF: So are there other reasons why you didn't call when you were feeling this way?

Janis: What do you mean?

GAF: That at a time when you felt so bad, so suicidal, that you chose not to call?

Janis: I couldn't. I told you it was hard . . . humiliating. *(As she sadly realizes her state of affairs, she sinks even deeper into the softness of the chair.)*

GAF: So it's death before revealing your need or vulnerability, even to me?

Janis: Jeez. You are a real pain in the ass. You never let up. You really like this work? People like me — fucked up, wasted, worried, weird people who can't get their shit

116

together . . . day after day you listen to this stuff. Jeez!

GAF: (*Janis will ultimately experience my calm, focused approach as soothing and helpful in reducing her confusion and despair.*) Mmnn.

Janis: What of it?

GAF: I see that by not calling me or Dr. Brau when you were in such a state, that you must have been saying forget it, it's too humiliating to call. Better to get wasted or get zonked. Don't let him know you're in trouble. He took off. The hell with him.

Janis: Well . . . you did. I know, I know, it's crazy. Jesus. (*Long silence.*) I was so down I couldn't make a move. Like I was in a dream, a nightmare. I know you have a right to take a vacation.

GAF: Despair and hopelessness. They discourage anything you do to manage your needs by making the dangers seem insurmountable, by confusing the real picture. By keeping you from calling.

Janis: Yeah. Why does that happen?

GAF: Perhaps they offer relief from the

117

struggle.

Janis: What's so bad about that? Death would be a relief.

GAF: Because at the same time you're courting death you're also seeking life.

Janis: Yeah, that's right. I'm guess I am a real pain in the ass to you, huh? How do you stand it, seeing people like me? Don't you feel like telling me to fuck off? *(Her face slowly breaks into a smile, now teasing and checking at the same time.)*

GAF: Are you feeling that way about yourself?

Janis: Yeah, most of the time I feel like shit.

GAF: Maybe you anticipate from me what you feel about yourself?

Janis: *(Long Silence)* No. I never really think of you as being . . . anything. Like you're . . not . . . like not judging. You, you're not . . . human—no I don't mean that, but it's as though you're not real . . . and super real at the same time. I don't know what I'm saying. Man this is hard. *(My reliability and consistency of attitude and response are critical to her sense of being real. As far as she is concerned, in me there will be one object in her life which she can experience as constant, and therefore real. This problem is not typical dependency. Janis functions quite independently. Rather, it is about having no feeling for her internal objects, no sense of them being here and real, so that she can have them when alone. Their absence leaves her alone to deal with the incoherent dread of the dead zone.)*

GAF: Both real and not real at the same time?

Janis: Yes, yes! It's all fucked up, doc. I get so confused, all I can think of is booze and smack and . . . and shit. *(Shakes her head)* I had a dream this morning, I mean actually it was more like, I'm not sure, maybe around one o'clock this afternoon, just before I woke. But it's like uh, I'm uh, I don't think . . . I want to tell you. It won't be mine anymore. It'll be gone. *(Here Janis reveals the tenuous nature of her connections to objects and to herself. The dream is part of her current self-experience and has become concretized as if it had physical existence. To reveal it is to give a part of her self away.)* I'm so tired, doc, just so tired. *(Long sigh)*

GAF: If you tell me it'll be gone? Why wouldn't it be that we would both have it? *(Such an idea doesn't often occur to her with respect to such deeply personal, inner experiences.)*

Janis: Oh! Gee that's cool, man. Yeah, we could share it, you think? Huh? Ya think? That'd be cool. Okay, okay. I was in some strange place, this was the dream. And it was weird, man—I mean the whole thing was weird. Outa sight. It was San Francisco, like out in Haight-Ashbury you know, my scene, man. There were a lot of people on the street walking around, socializing. I didn't know any of them. I talked to some of them and they didn't even look at me, they didn't even see me, *(In a squeaky, high pitched voice reflecting her tension)* Didn't even see me! That's my scene, my scene. I mean, jeez. How could they not know me? So I'm next to this . . . guy. I stand right in front of him. He looks at me and doesn't smile or anything. All of a sudden he turns into, uh, like a wizard, with a dark blue cape and hat and black eyes that could burn a hole through steel. But I'm curious and not afraid much. So I say something— hello I think. He doesn't say anything, just stares at me. *(Becoming very animated while recounting her dream, Janis begins to speak much faster, almost frenetically.)* Now I'm getting afraid, then I get angry and ask him what the fuck he's looking at. I don't know whether to get away or punch him. He still doesn't say anything and I'm confused. I reach over to touch his cape and my hand goes right through him, like he's a shadow, a silhouette or something . . . supernatural. I'm still calm now and I try to touch him again, and he becomes sticky, and I can't get free. My hand's pulled in, then my arm, and then I panic. It feels like I'm going to be . . . to sink into him. But as soon as I yank my hand back, I'm free. And he's still just, just standing there looking at me. And I'm not scared anymore. I woke up scared but then I wasn't. It was really weird, but I felt okay that day, for a while. So . . .what'd ya think? Am I crazy or what? *(Janis is on the edge of her seat.)*

GAF: When did you have this dream?

Janis: The night after I missed my appointment.

GAF: After your office called to cancel your appointment?

Janis: The next night. After you called to confirm today's appointment.

GAF: Uh huh. What comes to mind when you remember the dream?

Janis: I don't know. It was fucking wild. And scary. And way out. The wizard was one scary cat. I felt okay even though I was afraid. That doesn't make any sense does it? The scene — I don't get those people.

GAF: The people who didn't see you?

Janis: Yeah, man. How could they not see me? I know everybody in Haight-Ashbury, man.

GAF: How did you feel in the dream, when they didn't see you?

Janis: Hey, jeez! I don't know, it . . . that was a real bummer, man. They didn't even see me. I got distracted by the wizard, but they were like . . . almost like, uh . . . ghosts or something. But I thought to myself, in the dream, don't they know me, or are they snubbing me? Well, fuck them. And I was going to find somebody or something, I dunno, when I ran into the wizard.

GAF: Have you felt that way before, that you aren't being seen?

Janis: Yeah. (*slowly*) Sometimes I get pretty down when there's no one around or talking to me and I think, nobody gives a fuck, why is everybody down on me? I can't stand being ignored.

GAF: Uh huh. What comes to mind about the wizard?

Janis: That fuckin' wizard — ya know, his eyes were like pure black. Evil, but soft, too. I'm thinking evil, but then I also think . . . he was cool, man, like with the dark blue duds, and there was something softer in his eyes even though they were shiny black. The blue cape was like superman's in the comics, ya know? And when I went through his arm with my hand, I think I was more surprised than scared. No, I was scared too. At first I thought, he's gonna kill me. Then I thought, maybe he's friendly. Then that sticky shit, that was weird, I mean it was way out man. I was panicked. But it's funny, it didn't hurt or anything. But I was scared. Terrified. (*Clearly excited by this dreamwork, Janis awaits my comments with great anticipation.*)

GAF: Black, evil eyes?

Janis: Yeah, black and shiny. Sort of like yours. I thought that his eyes were evil, then I thought, soft, then I got confused. Now that I think of it, I felt a lot like I do in here sometimes. Oh, jeez, I just realized, for a moment in the dream I had this uh, I dunno . . . this idea flashed . . . that his eyes could see into my mind and that he knew everything about me. (*Brief silence.*) I think I wasn't sure whether to be scared or not.

GAF: And the dark blue?

Janis: I don't know. It was not too dark, more of a medium blue, just like the color of these chairs. Oh shit. The wizard — that's you, right? Jesus! I can't believe this stuff. Oh, I just had another flash. The wizard in his blue cape makes me think of you in the blue chair somehow. Jeez. I felt just as mixed up about him as I do about you. Am I right? Is that possible?

GAF: Mmmm. So everybody ignores you, but he bores in on you with his eyes?

Janis: Yeah, isn't that weird? Nobody

ignores me. I'm hard to ignore. My mother always said I needed a lot of attention when I was a kid. So I don't get why I should dream about not getting any. And that wizard. He was giving me plenty of attention and I guess now, looking at it, that I wasn't sure about him—not sure about. . . I don't know about what. I think there was a time in the dream I felt he was okay. But when my hand went through his arm, that was scary. I got all confused. (*Brief silence.*) And the stickiness—it was like I wouldn't be able to get loose, like I'd be pulled in and swallowed up. Jeez! The wizard, the wizard, he's you, man, he's you, isn't he? (*Stares off blankly*) I know it is. His eyes, he could see right through me. You . . . see right through me. Sometimes I am afraid of you just like I was of him. But I . . . you're not, you haven't done anything to make me afraid. Except I need you too much. I could just disappear, like whoosh, just like my hand going through his, your arm. (*Janis has once again described the need-fear dilemma. Her psychological-mindedness and ability to perceive the hidden meaning in the dream, for example, point to a more favorable prognosis.*) You're the only one who knows what's happening with me. Without you, I'm nothing, not real, like in the dream when nobody paid attention to me. They weren't ignoring me. I wasn't real, I wasn't really there to them. Only the wizard was there and I'd be alone without him. And I was sure he was there, but I was angry at him for scaring me. Then when I tried to touch him and went right through him, Jesus. Even he wasn't really there. And so I wasn't really there . . . or anywhere. Or maybe I was him when I touched him. I don't know . . . (*Silence)*

GAF: You're scared and angry at how much you depend on me. When I left on vacation, you became frightened at how alone you felt, how alienated from yourself and everyone else you felt, as in the dream when no one noticed you. You became enraged with me for abandoning you, and so you saw me as dark and evil and you decided to lash out at the wizard. But your lash turned into a touch because you also needed me and didn't want to destroy me. Then you feared that maybe I wasn't real, shown by your going right through me. So you expressed your rage by getting high and not coming to the first appointment on my return. (*Here I attempt to weave*

126

*the dream interpretation with her
reality to help put it together.)*

Janis: I'm really fucked up, huh? (She
seems *sad and subdued, but not for
very long.)* So how come I'm
fucked up like this? Why me,
huh? Why? *(more silence)* Ya
know, doc, I get so tired, so tired.
*(Janis looks depleted as she often does in
sessions. Although she rebounds at
other times, I have a sense that her
struggle with the deadness is pulling
her down. I am concerned that she
may not have the endurance for the
years of psychotherapy needed.)* I do
think that Jimi had it right . . . it's
just too hard, too fucking hard.
(Another brief silence.) Let me ask
you what you think. If you were
me, and you knew what you know
now, would you feel like, uh, cool,
like . . . hopeful? Come on, doc,
would you? Would you?
*(Desperately hoping for words that
would change the way she feels)*

GAF: Yes.

Janis: You'd say that anyway. Why yes?
Why? I can't make it through the
day without booze, smack, sex or
some other shit. My mind's all
messed up and I look like shit. I'm
fat and I can't hold onto anybody.
They all left. Everyday is

exhausting. I already feel dead. So why should I feel hopeful? Why? Dead seems like a pretty good idea—no more of this. So tell me why I should hope. *(Janis is truly feeling hopeful and hopeless at one and the same time. She is prodding me in an attempt to resolve her ambivalence.)*

GAF: Here is a good example of how you trap yourself in a no-way-out scenario. If I tell you there's hope, your hopelessness will not let you believe that I believe it. That's what hopelessness does: make us all disbelieve. If, on the other hand, I agree that it is hopeless, then your hopefulness will cause you to disbelieve. You try to keep away from either place— hope and hopelessness. The danger of hope or hopelessness is the same—they can both lead you closer to the same dreadful, avoid-at all-costs experience. Hopelessness can lead to death. But so can hope, because something in you seems to die everyday when you experience the overwhelming intensity of your human needs followed by the threat of abandonment and the terrifying nothingness when those needs aren't met. So you try to stay in between, that is, to stay in neither place, to stay nowhere.

Janis: (*Janis slumps more completely in the chair and looks at me. This bit of interpretation has caught her interest in that it seems to be an accurate description of something she feels but has never quite understood.*) Yeah, I do, I do. It's better than . . . (*She shakes her head and slowly begins to cry softly, unable to find words.*)

GAF: Better than . . .

Janis: I don't know. I read Sarte a long time ago. It left me feeling weird, like he knew something about me — the despair, the despair of life. He . . . it was about despair and I remember thinking then that it was about me, too. And you . . . you know even more about what's in my head. (*Long silence.*) Better? It's better than the . . . nothing . . . better than the confusion, better than the mess in my head. It's just that I can't stay there, keep away from despair for long. And I hate the longing, the need for love. It's too painful. Just as you said, everybody leaves and then it's . . . (*There is a perceptible shudder as Janis tries to describe the indescribable, the sense of annihilation which grips her in the face of object-connection failures. She cannot hold on to the connection to anyone. Her life forces are slowly being destroyed. Her will to be, to fight the forces of death and to value life is being depleted. She is slipping into the abyss. I am touched by her inability to feel life and at the same time feeling life so intensely that it overwhelms her with anxiety. She is not able to move between the extremes of emptiness and intensity and draw on both creatively, except perhaps when she is at her work. I fear for her survival.)*

GAF: Like death?

Janis: Worse! Where the fuck is everybody going? Why do they all leave? You can't count on anybody.

GAF: Perhaps you help people to leave.

Janis: What do you mean?

GAF: You've told me that some of your boyfriends left because they didn't like the way you fooled around with other guys, and that others didn't like your moods, the drinking and the drugs. If your goal was to have a close, intimate relationship, why didn't you adjust your behavior to get it?

Janis: Well shit, doc, I can't relate to that. I have to be true to my game, not theirs. I like having fun and doing what feels good. *(Janis now shifts emotions and actively begins to defend her behavior. As is often the case with borderlines of this sort, it's difficult for her to accept blame for her problems.)*

GAF: So you need or value the drugs, alcohol, and multiple partners more than a close, one-to-one relationship?

Janis: Jesus, why do you put it that way? I just have to do my own thing, man, that's all. Why are you blaming me? I can't help it if the cats are never there when you need them. You just can't trust them. They always let you down. *(Becoming more annoyed, and then sulking)*

GAF: So it's just the way it is? Your actions have little to do with all the disappointment you have about relationships? You're just a very unlucky chick?

Janis: Well, maybe I am a ballbuster sometimes. I just want people to be sincere and to have a good time. *(smiles proudly)* Some cats can't handle it.

GAF: Or maybe you feel threatened, as we've discussed before — fear of the intensity of your longing and the terror of being abandoned can cause you to short- circuit a relationship you may really want before you can feel the dread of being separated. Even a short separation from the person can cause you great anxiety once you become attached to them.

Janis: You think I sabotage relationships?

GAF: Don't you think so?

Janis: I don't know. I've never thought of it that way. I can relate to being needful. Sometimes when I need something, when I need to get down, man, I can get goin', get groovin' and nothing can stop me. Ya know? Like I can't stand being . . . like stopped.

GAF: When you're needy, you're impulsive and persistent?

Janis: Right. (*For borderline personalities, impulsivity is often a defense against anxiety.*)

GAF: Does that happen with people? That is, do you feel the need to act impulsively, for example, sexually, when you're with someone you're getting close to?

Janis: (*Slowly*) You mean like when I ball

some guy I just met while I'm in a relationship with someone else?

GAF: Yes. Doesn't that usually help to sabotage the relationship?

Janis: Yeah, (*somewhat glumly*) I guess so. I don't know. I mean, jeez, what . . . why is everything so hard? I just need a lot of action, man, that's all.

GAF: What are you feeling when you go looking for sexual liaisons while in the midst of a love affair?

Janis: I don't know. Just feel the need to pick up some new talent and get it on. (*Clearly annoyed and a bit confused, she wrinkles her brow.*)

GAF: Is it hard for you to understand why that behavior may damage an existing relationship?

Janis: I . . . no I guess not. It's just that I have such an appetite.

GAF: Could it be that you become apprehensive or agitated in some way and impulsively seek relief by distracting yourself with new stimulation?

Janis: Yeah, I get bored man. It's fucking boring sometimes.

GAF: What times?

Janis: I don't know, different times for chrissakes.

GAF: How about when someone you are close to leaves you for a while? Or just leaves the room when you're having a disagreement?

Janis: (*Ponders my question*) Well, yeah. Like when Seth took off last month after I got pissed at him. He just left and I went nuts. I stayed smashed for three days and balled my brains out. That what you mean?

GAF: What happened to you when he left? I mean, what was it like for you when he left before you got to drinking and so forth?

Janis: You mean right after?

GAF: Yes.

Janis I . . . I'm not sure. It just seemed as though I was completely alone, ya know what I mean—as though there wasn't anybody else.

GAF: How was that for you to feel?

Janis: It was horrible. I felt horrible and

. . . and panicked. *(For Janis, like others in the dead zone, when people are gone, they are gone – do not exist anymore, are not real.)* I couldn't stand it, just couldn't stand it, him just leaving like that.

GAF: Didn't you expect him to be angry at your behavior?

Janis: I don't know, I didn't think about it.

GAF: How come? *(I am working here to let Janis see the contradiction between her complaints that no one sticks around so that she is always lonely on the one hand, and her behaviors that are so destructive to intimate personal relationships on the other.)*

Janis: How come? I don't know, jeez. I guess.

GAF: Maybe we can discuss this further next time.

Janis: Fuck!

In these and hundreds of sessions to follow, Janis tries with great persistence to grasp the deadness and contain its effects on her personality. No one can predict the outcome, but if after a number of years (five to eight or more) she is to be able to organize a structured lifestyle and she uses the therapist as well as she has in these sessions, then her world might gain some measure of stability and peace. It is likely that her talents will remain intact and that a reasonably gratifying, "safe" relationship will develop. She will remain unpredictable and impulsive over the years, but nevertheless slowly improve her ability to control the torment of the dead zone.

Chapter Five: Jim Morrison - Poet, Shaman, Lizard King

I am the lizard king, I can do anything.

Like Janis, Jim was eventually destroyed by his inability to escape the dead zone; and like Janis he was far more than his searching, disharmonious and self-destructive impulses might suggest. Jim possessed a deeply intellectual and complex mind, capable of synthesizing wildly discordant experiences and ideas. He created a musical style that captured the universal longing for meaning that he hoped was hidden in the mystical, in the arcane. Unable to find relief from the alienation that was his constant companion, he sought escape through the chaos he experienced as maximum entropy. From that peculiar vantage point, the very existence of order and its accompanying rules blocked the opportunity to "break on through" the chaos he endured, and find the meaning that might have ended his despair.

The life of Jim Morrison has been amply chronicled in several books that have been most helpful to our study: *Break On Through* by James Riordan and Jerry Prochnicky, *No One Here Gets Out*

Alive by Jerry Hopkins and Danny Sugerman, and *Riders On The Storm* by John Densmore, the Doors' drummer. As we reviewed these and all the other material on Jim Morrison, we tried to look beyond the intellectual brilliance he frequently flashed through his weird and obnoxious behavior. All of his biographers presented a portrait of him as a taunting, teasing, hostile, oppositional man whose embrace of the dark side reflected his own deeply embedded despair and alienation. However much he repelled us, we could not help but be touched by the depth of his suffering, a suffering he tried to relieve with his heavy drinking, constant drug abuse and often sadistic behavior. Few passages from any biography were as painful to read and as revealing as this one from *Break On Through*:

> A diary of Jim's, thought to be from around this period (at the end of his life, in Paris), is riddled with a sense of helplessness — scrawled passages of desperation in lines like 'God help me, God help me, God help me' scribbled over and over again, filling entire pages. It is as though he cast away the last vestiges of caution, finally delving into the one substance that he had held back from before (Riodan and Prognicky 1991, 461).

But, of course, no one was really capable of helping him at that time.

Jim was raised in the south, in Florida, New Mexico and Washington, D.C. by his conventional middle class parents. They held to the societal values characteristic of the 1950's, were supportive of their progeny and encouraged their higher education. His biographers did not note any abuse, alcoholism or significant family disturbances. Like Janis', Jim's family consistently and patiently tried to understand and help, though Jim repeatedly rejected the basic values of his family.

Well read and possessing superior intelligence, Jim (like Janis) had read poets such as Corso, Ferlinghetti, McClure, and Jack Kerouac (Amburn 1992, 141). However, Jim was drawn to the more arcane, darker-toned literature of Plutarch, Baudelaire, Kafka, Rimbaud, Joyce, Balzac, Cocteau and Moliere. Jim was witty, quick, rebellious, oppositional and tended toward the outrageous.

Like Janis, Jim had no clear goals in mind when he graduated from high school. Although he finished school with good grades, he consistently underachieved, using only part of his intelligence, or using his intelligence inconsistently and unevenly. Jim appeared to have attained his rock star status as Janis did (see chapter three) by a confluence of unusual circumstances: the emerging, youthful, student counterculture of the sixties whose behaviors often "looked" just like those acted out by Jim, his own rapidly expanding interest in radically new life experiences, and the considerable artistic talent he possessed for developing music.

In L.A., Janis was known as "the female Jim Morrison," and in San Francisco, the *Doors* were known as "Hollywood's version of Big Brother," Janis' first group (Amburn 1992, 133). Jim, like Janis, used and continued to use drugs and alcohol until he died. He was a lost soul without a solid identity, could not sustain a mature adult relationship, died at 27 and lived the whole of his life in the dead zone.

Though similar in numerous ways, their lives could otherwise be characterized as different in one very significant aspect: their individual attempts to escape a dead inner world. Janis tried to escape by openly embracing hope, searching for affection, sensuality, eroticism, intense emotion. Her focus was on love and sex. That she was unable to assimilate all that she encountered had tragic, deadly consequences.

Jim, on the other hand, looked for an exit from his living hell by joining forces with darkness and destruction, by embracing the "other side" and seeking to "break on through" to another level of experience by out-deviling the devil. To that end he focused on sex and violence. Put differently, the same underlying forces that generated Janis' obsession with people, sex and life were the same forces that moved Jim to embrace demons, discord, and death.

Background

James Douglas (After General Douglas MacArthur) Morrison was born in 1943 to parents who were "kind, affable and upwardly mobile" (Riordan and Prochnicky 1991, 26). Jim's father was one of three children born in Florida to a conservative laundry owner. He was something of a goody-goody in high school and rather popular with the girls. He later saw action in World War II as a carrier pilot and in Korea where he coordinated carrier based air attacks, subsequently commanding an aircraft carrier and eventually being promoted to rear admiral (Hopkins and Sugerman 1980, 9).

Hopkins and Sugerman describe Morrison's mother as "one of five children of the slightly kooky, fun-loving daughter of a maverick lawyer from Wisconsin." She met Jim's father at a navy dance around the time the Japanese were preparing to bomb

Pearl Harbor. Riordan and Prochnicky claim that neighbors remember her as an "attractive, witty and active person who had a few oddities of her own." She is described as something of a nature lover and beachcomber, often using a metal detector. She wouldcollect sand dollars and sea shells used to craft home decorations.

Neither parent spanked the children (Jim had a younger brother and sister). Verbal admonitions were used instead. Away much of the time, Jim's father fluctuated between treating his children as recruits and exercising little parental authority, choosing instead to let his wife apply whatever discipline might be necessary.

Mr. Morrison's duty assignments forced his family to move from station to station: Jim lived in Pensacola, Melbourne, and Clearwater, Florida, twice in both Washington, D.C. and Albuquerque, New Mexico, and once each in Los Altos, Claremont, and Alameda, California before he finally attended high school in Alexandria, Virginia.

On the strength of that feature of Jim's background, some have suggested that this travelogue lifestyle and the absent father left too little structure in Jim's life and contributed to his problems as an adult. The frequent moves that are so much a part of military life can often create stress for a family. Perhaps it did for Jim, though his brother and sister appear to have emerged from that experience undamaged.

To say that Jim Morrison was a difficult child is to understate significantly what his biographers have written. Riordan and Prochnicky write that Jim "grew to be a minor terror within his family," a hell-raiser, demanding attention, causing much embarrassment, and resenting his siblings. Hopkins and Sugerman describe in every painful detail how Jim would physically and psychologically torment his brother, Andy (Hopkins and Sugerman, p. 30). Neither his sister nor his high school girlfriend escaped his sadism. In a pattern that continued throughout his short life, he mistreated and often abused his mother, the women he picked up, several girlfriends (including Janis Joplin) and his most enduring paramour, Pamela Courson.

Jim's intelligence apparently made it easy for him to be difficult and rebellious in school. He would not work consistently on assignments. He was perceived to be a "brilliant recluse," preferring instead to study unusual, abstruse, mystical subjects and historical figures. He spent some time researching information about reptiles, his fascination with them reaching a peak with his "I am the lizard king" pronouncement. He rejected conventional academic topics and authority of any kind. Instead he used his intelligence to produce extraordinary reports on strange, uncommon subjects. His biographers write of his early oppositional behavior, referring to such outrageous behaviors as yelling out "hey motherfucker" to passersby in the hall during the middle of a class, or giving outlandish excuses for tardiness (e.g., he had been robbed on the way or he had had an operation for a brain tumor). He delighted in challenging teachers with complex ideas and often used his wits to try to humiliate them. For example, he would delve deeply into unassigned but sophisticated readings and proceed to quiz his teachers. He constantly attempted one-ups-man-ship, believing himself to be smarter than they. Immersing himself in philosophy and existential literature, he was very familiar with figures such as Hume, Montaigne, Sartre, Nietzsche, Kafka, as well as Greek and Roman history, and he especially admired Alexander the Great. He was also fascinated by the pornographic, violent dime store novels he read constantly.

Jim is further described as an attention-seeking, sullen, rowdy, uncooperative, exceptionally intelligent loner who rejected the idea of being anything, and violently resisted conforming to conventional standards. In college he conducted himself as he did in high school. It wasn't long before his roommates asked him to leave because of his unrelenting self-centered, inconsiderate and exploitative behaviors, e.g., refusing to lower his loud music, taking others' clothes without permission, not carrying his share of the workload, and so on.

John Densmore writes about similar complaints and about how irresponsible Jim was before and during performances. The *Doors*, Ray Manzarek, John Densmore and Robby Krieger, were living on the edge in their association with Jim as much as they were in the music they played together. They felt as a group that they were unusual because the music they played was "on the edge" of acceptable music: spontaneous, raw and innovative. They created the music and the mood as they played, experiencing the intensity and breaking down old musical conventions. Morrison called the Doors "sexual politicians." They all accepted that term but invested it with a different meaning than Jim did. We doubt that they felt what Morrison felt. They used similar language but it referred to different inner experiences.

In college, Jim continued to pursue a wide variety of interests and often found himself drawn to the surrealistic. In keeping with his character, his tastes and interests shifted frequently, depending on what persona he was creating at the time. Jim was charismatic and could draw people into his game, manipulating them, all the while remaining quite detached from the hostile feelings he generated in others. His early years were prologue to the search that consumed his energies afterward and eventually destroyed him—the search for a self and for meaning, for a way to break through his merciless despair.

Break On Through: Embracing The Dead Zone

Like Janis, Jim used alcohol, drugs and sex in every way he could. He was persistent, and, unlike Janis, sadistic. Some have said that in these pursuits Jim was actually testing the bounds of reality and reminding us where the name "Doors" came from. Morrison was taken with a line from William Blake: "If the doors of perception were cleansed every thing would appear as it is, infinite."

Jim's biographers report that he used to quote Blake, "There are things known and unknown and in between are the doors". Aldous Huxley had taken the Blake line and written *The Doors of Perception,* telling of his own attempts to find new levels of mind and consciousness through the use of mescaline. The idea of skirting the edge, of breaking down convention and gaining a cleansed perspective, appears to have captured that part of Jim which sought to escape the dead zone by "knowing" the mystical and the visionary. In seeking the mystical and the visionary, he sought to "understand the relationship of words to things, of systematic reasoning to the unfathomable mystery which it tries, forever vainly, to comprehend" (Huxley as cited in Hopkins and Sugerman, 45).

Given these propensities, it is not surprising that Jim was drawn to the darker poets and writers such as Edgar Allen Poe, Franz Kafka and especially Arthur Rimbaud. From surrealism, Morrison quickly adopted the notion of reaching into the subconscious and disorder to find order, into illusion to find reality. Rimbaud moved these surrealistic ideas to even greater extremes by seeking the logical through the illogical and sanity through insanity. Jim also talked of pursuing sanity through insanity, and so he embraced the arcane, the hidden, the mysterious, the inscrutable, the extreme, the illogical, the disordered and the sensual (Riordan and Prochnichy, 134). How else could any true understanding take place?

Thus Jim constantly lived on the edge, captured by the lure of escape which he thought that mode of living would offer. Sharing that state of mind with him, *The Doors* performed and lived on the narrow border between the rational and the irrational, the real and the surreal, the known and the unknown.

Jim's efforts to break through the limits of the senses and ordinary experience were not driven by intellectual forces or curiosity, but by the irresistible dread emanating from an inner place most of us will never know. Everyone who has written about him has made it clear that Jim drank heavily, not for enjoyment but to get drunk. Like Janis, he tried many drugs but eventually settled on heroin. We do not find this surprising because as we noted earlier, both alcohol and heroin obliterate awareness of pain. In spite of the many attempts to escape that terrible destination, the lives of these two artists were overwhelmed by the same dread.

The purpose of Jim's self-destructive substance abuse was not to discover the other side but to *escape* to the other side. He sought to escape the deeply distressing anxiety emanating from an inner world more lonely for him than if he had grown up somehow without human contact. By behaving in an outrageous and provocative manner, Jim attempted to fill the void, to prevent panic from overwhelming him. Hanging off the ledge of a tall building, rambling on in a trance like a shaman, cursing his audience, instigating a police officer to arrest him, tormenting a bus driver or a teacher were all actions driven by the same demons. And they were the same demons that plagued Janis. The greater the tension he could generate in the world because of his actions, the less he felt the alienation, despair and dread.

Riordan and Prochnicky discuss Jim's antics this way:

> . . . he never did them for publicity. He did them for excitement. He got in barroom brawls. He swung nude from the bell tower at Yale. He played matador with the cars on the freeway. He challenged cops repeatedly and was maced, clubbed, and beaten more than once (Riordan and Prognicky, 234).

Hopkins and Sugerman write that he was "by his own admission attracted to extremes." They quote Jim as saying, "I think the highest and lowest points are the important ones. All the points in between are, well, in between. I want freedom to try everything—I guess to experience everything at least once."

As with Janis, however, the real motive, for this tragic pattern of excitement-seeking was by no means clear to him. That is, Jim and Janis may have been aware of the desire to provoke or create some havoc around them, to experience everything, but they were unaware of the deeper forces and motives propelling them. Janis said she was just an unconventional type who saw through the hypocrisy of many social values and was doing her own thing. Jim intellectualized and justified his actions by espousing a search for knowledge beyond the realm of the common, into the subconscious, seeking to learn from chaos. Whatever explanation Jim may have attached to his behavior, there is overwhelming evidence that his exploration of the other side was a very complex effort of an intelligent but troubled mind to solve a problem: that of living a life without internal objects. Life without experiencing internal objects is living a life in utter desolation. We can only feel "real" when we have the capacity to experience the presence of early significant others within ourselves. Without the essential experience of 'realness' that comes from feeling oneself to be connected to those internal objects, anyone would experience an intolerable existential despair.

Jim Morrison was once quoted as saying that he felt his imagination was liberated onstage, and Ray Manzarek observes:

> For Jim, being onstage was just about everything. On stage he came alive and was the most exciting and dynamic performer I'd ever seen. He would go through trips onstage . . . you wouldn't believe the personalities that would come out of him, the intensity that he would speak to the audience (Riordan and Prochnicky, 187).

But perhaps Riordan and Prochnicky themselves offer the best characterization of his performances:

> Watching him sing was like witnessing a man dangling in his own anguish. Seeing him scream, writhe, and whisper his way into a head-on clash with some ultimate truth in song could be truly frightening.

Even the most unfeeling in the audience sensed that the sudden shrieks and violent screams came from somewhere deep within the subconscious. (Riordan and Prochnicky, p. 186)

Morrison acted out on many levels. Not all were entertaining; few were understood. Morrison could ponder the mystical, experiment with concepts, dabble with the notion of creative chaos, and write surreal poetry. But he was a Jekyll and Hyde character— unpredictable, self-destructive and confused. His alienation from others and from himself was complete, and he experienced it practically from the beginning.

Searching For Jim: Lost Between The Doors

The Shaman

Jim Morrison quit the Doors, we believe, to find himself, to become a person with a solid, continuous self-feeling, to continue the struggle with his increasing alienation from life itself. He needed to find a self. How could he have known that the common developmental task we all face would be forever impossible for him? He knew something was wrong. Before he left to live the remaining months of his life in Paris, he said, "I don't know who I am, I don't know what I'm doing, I don't know what I wanna do . . . I'm gone . . . don't count on me, goodbye." Neither the instigative, thrill-seeking, chaotic, outrageous behaviors, nor the fine intellect and talent could rescue him from the dead zone. His vulnerability to the splitting of experience and to object inconstancy frustrated all his efforts to feel real and stable, to feel okay, and to feel himself to be the same person continuously from moment to moment.

Jim had always sought self-definition. This search was marked first by constant attention-seeking as a child. When he still couldn't feel his own existence, he then looked to others for the reactions and responses he needed to bolster himself and to derive something of a sense of self, however vague and shifting. His troublesome childhood behaviors foreshadowed adolescent and adult misadventures and stimulus seeking. As an adult, he pressed his intellect into serving his search for a solid self. His futile attempts to fashion a "me" for himself included displays of intellectual arrogance, preoccupation with bizarre and esoteric subject matter, and the presentation of an oppositional, I'm-different-from-everyone-else attitude.

Eventually, Jim tried to fit himself into a life role, hoping to find the self he had always been looking for. Of course, this role had to be intense and special. Only by passing through the doors of perception into the mystical and the unconventional—outside of the world in which he found no solace—might he find himself. Hence his shamanism. And his poetry. And the lizard king.

Much has been made of the incident he witnessed as a child where a truckload of Indians had been injured and killed in an accident. As the medicine man lay dying on the side of the road, his spirit, it is alleged, had entered Jim's body. Though our analysis suggests that we shouldn't attribute very much of anything to that accident, Jim did eventually come to see himself as a shaman, as having the special power to see through the falsehoods of this world into the next, to that world beyond the "doors of perception." According to this rather unconventional account of how Jim came to be the bizarre character he was, people become shamans by experiencing a close call with death or some other deadly trauma. This is followed by rebirth, and then instruction regarding the spirit world is given. Shamans thereafter deal in dreams, visions, reveries, trances, mythology and spirits. As unique spirits, they can be moody, irritable, depressed and anxious, as well as emotionally hyper-reactive and isolative.

This occult-like identity fit Jim's needs for a time, and he reveled in it. He began trying on the identity of a "rock shaman." One article called him "a slithering sorcerer" in response to his shamanist leanings and famous "I am the lizard king" pronouncements. Jim proposed that his performances helped him do what shamans do: relieve the sickness of others by taking on their evil urges and becoming evil's repository. He claimed that by entering into trances onstage he enhanced the shamanic process. Doors' audiences were moved by the arcane and intensely emotional quality of these shamanist rituals, especially when combined with rock music and Morrison's stage presence. How Jim understood himself as he conducted these concerted exercises in emotional tension while instigating chaos was perhaps best summed up in a quote about such a role:

> I am possessed by the spirit of a shaman.
> I see the role of the artist as shaman and
> scapegoat. People project their fantasies
> on to him and their fantasies come alive.
> By attacking and punishing me people
> can feel relieved of their impulses.
> (Riordan and Prochnicky, p. 192)

In our view, it wasn't the fans who needed to be

relieved of their impulses. Failing to recognize the need in himself, Jim projected that need onto the everyone else. The audiences' reactions were meant to shore up his failing self and prevent his disintegration of self-feeling. How could he have known that he was squandering his psychological resources on the search for his substance, for a feeling of existence, for that nebulous entity called a self?

That search turns out to be mostly hopeless for those who live in the dead zone. Whether one refers to it as the "I", the "me", "identity", the "core self", or the "self organization", Jim had no experience of it. He was really a man without a center. He couldn't find his way based on any internal compass because the one normally used—that abstraction we routinely label "me"—did not exist for him. His core self (which is created out of the experience of one's own existence) had never been formed. It was lost or unfinished, floating somewhere between the doors of perception, between the known and the unknown.

The Poet

Poets attempt to move people by communicating at both the conscious and the unconscious level with the audience, presenting their own versions of the meaning of life and death by using language in an uncommon fashion. Jim had often declared himself a poet and he wrote throughout his short life. Several volumes of his work have been published since his death. His poetry failed to define him, however. His final notes of despair cited earlier make it quite clear that an integrated sense of self forever eluded him.

That this man of superior intelligence and talent

did not find himself in poetry was just another of the tragedies that befell him. From both a literary and a clinical point of view, there is no meaning to be found in Jim's poetry nor in his attempt at film- making in college. His poetry and film seem to be a conglomerate of images of sex and death, images of a primitive, erotic, religious, chaotic and exotic nature. They are not integrated images and are without recognizable meaning. They seem to have been created out of the distorted fantasies and fragmentary shifting elements of a mind living in its own hell. The poetry, like the shamanism, was created for dual purposes: to stimulate a feeling of life and to organize an atomized and disordered collection of experiences into something resembling an identity.

Jim Morrison's poems can be widely interpreted, not because they are a synthesis of complex ideas and experiences, but rather because they are essentially without meaning except for the tormented confusion they reveal about the mind of the poet himself. His intelligence could not truly help him in this effort, though it did enable him to create a poet's facade as an identity, a "false self" which could only disintegrate from the moment it was constructed. That this was inevitable should not surprise us, since identities do not evolve out of whole cloth. They emerge slowly through internalization of the elements of those personalities, those significant people in one's early environment. These elements are then "metabolized" in the formation of the real self.

From the very beginning, Jim's vulnerability to splitting and object inconstancy limited his capacity to internalize the essence of significant others. In other words, he could not psychologically absorb all of the disparate experiences he so aggressively sought into a real self because he hadn't been able to internalize the essence of his parents as a child. The experiences had no place to go, no place where they could be taken and assimilated as part of an already developing self. No matter how many poems he wrote, trances he fell into, or images he provoked in his audiences, he was unable to use any of it. There was a black hole where self-feeling was supposed to be.

The Lizard King

Jim began his fascination and learned extensively about reptiles as a child. Later as a rock star he called himself the lizard king. Since reptiles commonly evoke fear and a sense of the mysterious, it seems clear that Jim was again drawn to the unusual and the occult in summoning the power of reptiles to induce strong reactions. The darker motivations of man are often ascribed to the "reptilian period" of man's evolution. This inscrutable quality of the reptile was a natural attraction for Jim. He projected his own hopes and fantasies into a reptilian identity, an identity he tried to feel by wearing the lizard skin suit he had made for himself. No one who saw him wearing that suit in concert will ever forget it.

In his reptilian rapture we might imagine him to be inspired by the imagery of being powerful, scary, and specifically—some kind of reality for himself— dark, dangerous and defined. His lizard suit reinforced his sense of *being*—someone whose presence he hoped to feel. "I am the lizard king " he said over and over again. Regrettably, the unfinished half of that pronouncement which Jim Morrison could not understand was "therefore I am." Tragically, unlike most adolescents who develop normally, he never could answer the question, "Who am I?" But then, few in the dead zone can.

These three pseudo-identities failed to catalyze the identity formation process. Jim desperately needed the emotional stability and soothing that should normally have occurred with the "metabolizing" of the raw materials of personality taken from those childhood caregivers who loved him and related to him. He was without any means of comprehending or preventing his demise. Splitting and object inconstancy, however they happen, are neither readily understandable nor easily treated.

Love Me Two Times: I Can't See Your Face In My Mind

Hopkins and Sugerman write of a phone call from Jim's mother. The Morrisons had not heard from their son for a very long time and were trying to locate him. A friend of Jim's brother, Andy, had been listening to a Doors album and recognized Jim's picture on the cover. His mother had called Elektra Records and convinced them that she was indeed his mother, thereby obtaining his phone number. Hopkins and Sugerman record the following conversation:

> Mrs. Morrison: Hello? This is Mrs. Morrison,
> is Jim there?
> Jim: Jim who?
> Mrs. Morrison: Jim. Jim Morrison. I'm his
> mother.
> Jim: Yeah? *(The man sounded bored.)*
> *(Another voice came on the line.)* Hello?
> Mrs. Morrison: Jim? Oh Jim . . .
> Jim: Yes, Mother . . .

He replied with a series of grunts and moans to his mother's concerns about his not calling, writing or even letting them know where he was and that he was all right. She asked him to come home for Thanksgiving dinner with the family. She asked him to get a haircut for his father's sake (now Admiral Morrison). He sighed and promised nothing. The others in the room were just listening. Hopkins and Sugerman record that Jim hung up and then said, "I don't want to talk to her ever again."

Jim had once told a reporter upon questioning that his parents were dead. They obviously weren't, and indeed some of those in the room must have been startled by this phone call from his mother. To Jim, who had great difficulty with object constancy—his parents were not internalized—they were in his memory but without any sense of realness, nor feeling of attachment. Therefore it was as though they did not exist for him. And because he couldn't feel their existence (in the sense described earlier), he couldn't feel his own.

Ironically, the title of one of his songs, "I can't see your face in my mind," reflects his vulnerability to object inconstancy. He simply could not bring to his mind any "emotionally valuable representation" of these early significant people in his life. Most likely, people were experienced by Jim as "objects," lifeless and unreal. Without such a capacity for object relations, he might as well have been living alone on Mars. He could not stay connected to anyone except briefly under conditions of extreme tension or stimulation. We see this in his interaction with all women, including Pamela Courson and Patricia Kennealy.

During his career with the Doors and up until

his death, Jim Morrison maintained a "relationship" with Pamela Courson. He had many other liaisons but always returned to her, and she seems to have treated him in kind. It would take a certain kind of partner to tolerate Jim's destructive behaviors. In startling detail, Riordan and Prochnicky describe (as told by Paul Rothchild, the Doors ' producer) the typical nature of his relationships with women in his encounter with Janis Joplin:

> She saw this hunk of meat (Jim) and said, 'I want that.' Jim would get drunk most days and this was no exception and as usual he got rude, obnoxious, and violent. He turned into a cretin, a disgusting drunk. And Janis who was a charming drunk, was really put off by him. Well the more Janis rejected him, the more he loved it. This was a kind of match. Janis finally said to me, 'let's get out of here,' and we went to the band station wagon that she always drove. Jim came staggering over. He reached into the car and started to say something and she told him to fuck off. She wasn't interested anymore. Jim wasn't going to take no for an answer, though, and he reached into the car and grabbed Janis by the hair. Well, she picked up a bottle of Southern Comfort she had, reached out of the car, and wailed him on the head with it. He was out cold. The next day, I saw Jim in rehearsal and he said to me, 'What a great woman. She's terrific. Can I have her telephone number?' He was in love. Physical confrontation was his thing. He

loved violence. (Riordan and Prochnicky, p. 173)

Riordan and Prochnicky also recount a typical incident that occurred with Pamela Courson. Frequently Pam and Jim argued about Pam wanting him to spend a quiet evening at home versus his wanting to party with friends. Often these arguments turned into knockdown, drag-out fights with their place getting smashed up despite all the careful work Pam had done in selecting furniture and decorating their apartment. This time after arguing:

> Pam began screaming at him to leave and take his junk with him and started hurling books and dishes in a full on barrage. Morrison scrambled out the door and made it downstairs without getting hit. Once he was in the clear, Pam began heaving his stuff out the window and a huge pile of books, clothes and records was soon strewn about the front lawn . . . . The next day, when he had sobered up and she had calmed down, they went out on the lawn, picked everything up, and resumed their life as if nothing had happened (Riordan and Prochnicky, 230).

This appears to us to be a revealing example of the instability in all his relationships, i.e. the creation of chaos and the inability to experience even a close partner as real, whole and satisfying for awhile. Ever since childhood Jim had reacted to his partners as a Jekyll and Hyde, sometimes gentle and charming, other times hostile, sadistic and destructive. This behavior is typical of the disturbed object relations of someone who cannot help but split the people with whom he is trying to connect with into partial beings without "realness." Such a person is unable to maintain object constancy. Such relationships are typical for those with a 'void' in place of a self.

When The Music's Over

> Before I sink, into the big sleep,
> I want to hear, I want to hear,
> The scream of the butterfly.

Twenty years after Jim Morrison's death, Densmore wrote that in the movie *The Doors*, actor Val Kilmer "miraculously re-created Jim." Densmore appears to have written his book as a modest attempt to comprehend his experience with the Doors and especially with the unpredictable, enraging and enigmatic Morrison. Densmore's observation that the movie accurately captured the tormented but outrageous Morrison is consistent with the analysis we are offering. For most of his life, Morrison gave a whole new meaning to the terms self-destructive, confused and desperate — symptoms of the borderline condition. Yet another instance in which art imitates life.

Like Janis, Jim had no true sense of himself. Like her, he was a talented performer in search of a self, ultimately losing his struggle with the demons of the dead zone. And like her he acted provocatively, impulsively and in accord with the need-fear dilemma (as described earlier, a primitive set of needs for nurturance and attachment counterbalanced by an equally primitive fear of closeness as threatening to one's own existence). They functioned inconsistently, had no center, no focus and no capacity to self-soothe, and thus couldn't handle the ever present but incoherent dread. Both sought to commune with their audiences, but Jim's hostility and sadism dominated his relationships with the audience and with women. Janis looked for love among the living to escape the dead zone, while Jim sought pain and death for the same reason. Densmore discovered a never-released interview with Jim by a Lizzie Smith in which Jim says:

> Pain is meant to wake us up. People try
> to hide their pain. But they're wrong.
> Pain is something you carry, like a radio.
> You feel your strength in the experience
> of pain. . . But people fear death even
> more than pain. It's strange that they fear
> death. Life hurts a lot more than death.
> At the point of death, the pain is over. I
> guess it is a friend (Densmore, p. 196).

Jim believed that life hurt more than death because of the unbearable quality of the only life he knew. Despairing and hopeless, those who live with borderline disorders are so drained of emotional resources that they almost always live with the thought of suicide or experience suicidal ideation every day. The consequences of having one's resources drained are constant existential despair and feelings of meaninglessness. Unable as he was to create the "internal objects" we all need in childhood, Morrison felt worse than dead. Riordan and Prochnicky:

> By the time of his death Morrison already
> knew that the real things tormenting him
> would not change with a new identity.
> He had a taste of that in Paris and

160

discovered that it didn't matter where he lived, how famous he was, or what kind of work he did. The problem had to do with the way he was inside . . It was his inability to cope with the forces inside him that was destroying him. The tormenting echoes that drove him to the brink of madness on an almost daily basis (Riordan and Prochnicky, 471).

So even Jim at some point and at some level understood the futility of fighting the good fight against an enemy that was as yet undefined and extremely lethal. That he was able to perform at all, let alone in the high intensity light emanating from the rock music world, is remarkable. Regrettably, the great majority of those who experienced his performances never really understood his motivations that lay just beneath the surface.

Jim: After All

We believe that Jim sadistically provoked people because he could only experience others (or himself) as not-quite-real "partial objects." His provocativeness, his instigation of the audience, and his lifelong sadism should be viewed as desperate attempts to kindle a fire in others intense enough to warm his own bitter cold soul. If he could incite others to high enough levels of emotional intensity, then he might experience them—and thus himself—as real. He would escape from the dead zone on the feelings of life from those whom he aroused to a fever pitch. His provocative behaviors toward his audiences and toward individuals, such as his obnoxious teasing of

Janis on their only encounter, are less confusing when understood in this way. Strong reactions from others gave him brief moments of escape.

Jim's life of intensely self-destructive abandon and hopelessness are familiar to clinicians who have worked with the identity diffused, emotionally isolative, or detached and internally barren patient. Based on our current clinical understanding of psychology and personality, we are now able to answer the same questions about Jim that we have already answered about Janis.

1. What was the matter with him? Why was his life such a chaotic affair?

The information we have gathered for this book, those observations of him made by his biographers, the portrayal of him in films, and his own words as recorded in personal interviews lead us to respond, as with Janis, to the two most frequently asked questions since his death.

To respond effectively, we must identify the characteristic features of Jim's' personality that permit us to offer our particular diagnosis. It is very clear to us now that (like Janis) he consistently exhibited:

- a clear pattern of instability in interpersonal relationships;
- an unstable and vague self-image and identity;
- shifting and unpredictable moods;
- a poor control of impulses and emotions beginning in early adulthood and evident in a variety of contexts.
- a pervasive feeling of emptiness/deadness

This description happens to be consistent with the same diagnosis we believe to have been the case for Janis: *Borderline Personality Disorder* as defined by the *Diagnostic and Statistical Manual of the American Psychiatric Association* (DSMIV, see appendix I).

Once again as with Janis, we can say that in modern clinical terms, the response to the first question is that Jim was increasingly incapacitated by a personality disorder that was little known or understood at that time. His chaotic life, like Janis', may now be understood as having resulted from that disorder. Typically, in their desperation to escape the inner feelings of tension and dread, most detached type borderline personalities like Jim tend to cut a confusing life path, interacting with others in complicated, intense yet superficial ways. Paradoxically, in their emptiness, detached types stay emotionally disconnected from life behind the numbing wall created by an objectless internal world. People we may know or read about who display many of the characteristics of Jim Morrison may well be struggling with borderline disorders.

2. How did he die? Did he kill himself?

We obviously can never know for certain. Pamela Courson arranged for his burial in Pere Lachaise cemetery in Paris before his death was made public. The only evidence available does not permit us to determine whether he deliberately killed himself or was simply another unlucky drug user. However, the question remains -why did he use drugs? We believe he took them to help manage the despair and the unbearable inner tension which were laying waste to his emotional life.

If his death (and Janis') was not an intentional suicide, it nevertheless came as a consequence of engaging in behaviors aimed at escaping the inner emotional barrenness of life. In a sense, Jim and Janis are examples of one kind of deadly conflict waged for the soul of a person, a conflict Karl Menninger described almost three decades ago in his book, *Man Against Himself.*

What Menninger concludes is that inexplicable external behaviors are the result of struggles with untamed, internal and aggressive forces present in all humans. These self-destructive and aggressive forces can be avoided only if one has achieved some form of psychological homeostasis via psychological mechanisms such as *sublimation, instinctual regulation,* and *personality integration.* The idea is that these psychological mechanisms develop from experiencing in one's childhood what is labeled a "good enough environment." Also needed is a temperament low in vulnerability to ordinary childhood stress (good protoplasm).

3. How was he different if at all from the many other public figures who died prematurely by their own hand?

Once again, as we asserted in chapter 3, there are probably other public figures who suffer with one of the many types of borderline conditions. But they are fewer in number compared to non-public individuals with the disorder. Clinicians at present are certain enough of the borderline profiles that they can easily point to Zelda Fitzgerald and Marilyn Monroe as possible borderline types. Monroe's biographers record chronic behaviors that are consistent with what we know today to be borderline conditions. Clinical psychiatry had not yet framed the outlines of the borderline disorder and so no one, including these celebrities, could find treatment for the condition, no relief from the dread.

Janis and Jim were unlike most public figures who die by their own hand. Many borderline patients who die this way, i.e. indirectly as an unintended outcome of the self-destructive nature of borderline conditions, are typically unable to become very public figures. Although there are many successful people struggling with a borderline condition, they tend toward a milder form of the disorder. As we noted in chapter 3, a moderate-to-severe borderline condition makes it difficult for someone to become a celebrity, except perhaps when public recognition is achieved by sensational behaviors.

Chapter Six: Reflections on Destiny: Jim in Therapy

I wish clean death would come to me

Joyce McDougall, the French psychoanalyst who has worked extensively with creative people of all types including those in the performing arts, believes that truly creative acts come not from whatever psychopathology an artist might have but from the healthiest part of the artist's personality. Like Janis, Jim was more than the sum of his psychological disturbances. Certainly the signs and symptoms of Jim Morrison's pathology covered the rock landscape. Nevertheless, his vocalizations, charisma, stage presence, songs, and some of his poetry emerged from the healthier elements in Jim's personality and did not derive from his borderline condition. The tragedy was that the full promise of Jim Morrison was unrealized at the time of his death.

Our contention is that Jim's reaction to a lifelong residency in the dead zone is the most reasonable explanation for his preoccupation with mystical ideas, madness, pain, chaos and death. He used his considerable intellect to try to batter his way out, and for the same reason was drawn to the writings of his intellectual mentors, Rimbaud, Blake, Nietzsche, and Kafka. They seemed to whisper in his ear: defy all conventional logic, stir up the pot, test all limits, flirt with the very edge of experience and beyond. Wasn't it Rimbaud who glorified madness, Blake who urged an alteration of perception, and Kafka who told of alienation from the self? Wasn't it Nietzsche who talked of supermen and of who saw a morality "beyond good and evil?" These were the intellectual ideas that informed Morrison's behavior.

Those who would glorify Jim's aberrant, outrageous and inane behaviors as the wellsprings of his creative process misunderstand him. The idea that Jim's behavior was the result of an intellectual journey of any kind is insupportable. Instead, his search for ways out of the dead zone caused him, like so many others, to seek the excitement of intense experiences, to escape the emptiness and inner chaos, and along the way to find the intellectual rationalization for his actions. That he was able to use his readings and philosophical explorations to create new combinations of words and themes in music and poetry is a tribute to his intelligence and the healthy side of him. He was creative in spite of his life in the dead zone, not because of it.

In their book, *No One Here Gets Out Alive,* Hopkins and Sugerman describe Jim's manipulation of the audience, teasing and waiting until they became restless and angry at his doing nothing, just standing in a trance, as he often did:

> It's like watching a mural . . . There's movement and then it's frozen. I like to

see just how long they can stand it, and
when they're about to crack, I let go
(Hopkins and Sugerman, 134).

Morrison was then asked about what he would do if
the crowd went berserk and rushed the stage like they
were going to kill him. He cited theories about the
sexual neuroses of crowds and then said:

I always know exactly when to do it.
That excites people. You know what
happens. They get frightened, and fear is
very exciting. People like to get scared.
It's exactly like the moment before you
have an orgasm. Everybody wants that.
It's a peaking experience. (Riordan and
Prochnicky 1991).

Of course, not everybody is like that, seeking the
ultimate thrill in defying danger or death. Indeed, it
appears his fans understood very little of the real
motivations for his antics.

While he was busy defying, Jim accumulated
quite an arrest record in the brief period of his adult
life. FBI records show him to have been arrested at
least ten times between 1963 and 1969 on such charges
as drunk driving, lewd and lascivious behavior,
battery, driving without a license, and interference
with the flight of an aircraft (Riordan and Prochnicky,
346-347). Consider how Jim's life might have turned
out if a judge, given this record, had ordered him to
undertake individual psychotherapy for alcohol abuse
while he was on probation.

Though there is little reason to believe that he
would have sought such help, Riordan and Prochnicky
report that Jim, on the urging of Pamela Courson's

father, once had a few sessions with a psychiatrist (Riordan and Prochnicky, 172). However, he played games with the psychiatrist, plying him with a stream of intellectual and philosophical gibberish, and then ending the sessions abruptly when he became bored. Simply forcing Jim into treatment with a competent therapist trained in borderline psychopathology may or may not have made a difference. Although Jim did not permit any serious analysis of his behavior and personality, we can offer an account of how a few sessions with Jim might have been.

Imagine then, a reluctant Jim Morrison ordered into psychotherapy, a common experience these days. The time is November, 1970. Following Jimi Hendricks by two weeks, Janis Joplin had died of complications following an injection of heroin. Jim is aware that he is slipping into despair, voicing his concern that he doesn't know who he is. The excitement of performing and inciting people isn't enough to quiet the demons anymore. At best the emptiness has become more dreadful. His first line of defense — alcohol — has ceased to numb the pain of the emptiness. He is thinking of getting away, thinking again of doing more work on his poetry. In his mind, Paris offers him hope as he plans to leave the Doors. Janis's death bothers him. He has his own lingering preoccupation with death. What follows are imaginary segments of several sessions conducted across many months in late 1970 and early 1971.

He reacts to psychotherapy with disdain and scorn, but he aches deep in his porous self-core and harbors a vague, unconscious hope that something or someone might pull him up from the void.

Session 1:

169

The first appointment occurs in late November, 1970. His long-suffering girlfriend Pam is to leave for Paris in February of 1971, and it is expected that he would follow her in April. The other members of the Doors had sensed Jim's restlessness and uncertainty about the future. So when he is ordered into treatment they are hopeful.

Jim shows up ten minutes late for the first appointment, overweight and bearded. I greet him. He looks around as he enters the room, avoids a handshake and sits without a word, waiting for me to start. He presents as cynical and detached, and has a strange, trance-like expression on his face, similar to the way he looks in the publicity pictures of him. He does not rush in to engage. I begin by explaining what I have been told about him:

GAF: My understanding is that you have been in some difficulty with the law. The probation officer told me you have been arrested on a number of occasions for various offenses, for driving while intoxicated and for lascivious behavior. In this last instance the judge ordered you to try six sessions of therapy as a condition of probation.

Jim: Yeah. *(Looking bored, he is dressed in tight black leather pants and a loose, white linen shirt. His face is drawn, perhaps from drugs or alcohol, and he is overweight. His dark, curly hair is rather unkempt. Slumped in his chair, leg sprawled, Jim doesn't look much like the young lion in the famous poster of him.)*

GAF: Can you enlighten me a bit about all this?

Jim: *(He is looking mildly annoyed and as though he is trying to decide whether to bother, but he finally does, speaking slowly and sarcastically without intonation.)* The uptight little man judge thinks he knows what he's doing but he doesn't. He doesn't get what it's all about and neither do you. What really matters isn't what he thinks matters, and he can't figure it out. It's not his fault he can't understand. He's hopelessly out of touch so he can't take it all in. *(Jim's intellectual arrogance is the by-product of using his mind to defend against the dread which always grips him.)*

GAF: How do you mean 'what really matters?'

Jim: *(Looking disinterested and speaking in monotone)* I'm not interested in this game . . . in your mindless shrink games. There's no point talking to you. You want to get into my mind, do your thing. Figure out why I do what I do. It's pointless. You can't. *(So far, Jim has used words/phrases such as, "can't figure it*

*out," can't understand," "hopeless,"
and "pointless." The words used by a
patient are important in that they often
apply elsewhere in his/her psychology.
Here I begin to wonder if Jim is feeling
hopeless too. I make a mental note of
this and of the possibility that his
history of drug and alcohol abuse is an
attempt at self-medication.)*

GAF: Well, maybe we could try anyway.

Jim: Maybe. (*Looking at me out of the
corner of his eye, one brow raised*) But
you don't seem any smarter than
the judge. Stuck here in your dull
little world.

GAF: (*Ignoring the hostility for now and
bringing in the reality of his situation*)
Well, it seems that the court is
requiring that you be in therapy
somewhere until your probation is
up. So as long as you're here,
maybe we can both learn
something instead of staring at
each other for fifty minutes.

Jim: Yeah . . . maybe. So what are you,
Freudian . . . Adlerian . . . Jungian?
(*Drifting off, he responds laconically. I
get little suspicious that he might be
high. His awareness of Freud, Adler,
and Jung reflect his reported familiarity
with some psychoanalytic literature.*)

GAF: Is it important to you which?

Jim: No, it doesn't matter.

GAF: What does matter?

Jim: *(Speaking softly, slowly and as if to himself)* Pain matters, chaos matters, death matters, sex matters, the senses matter, experiences matter . . . fear matters . . . the only realities.

GAF: Sounds a bit morbid.

Jim: *(Again, slowly and softly. I believe now that he has had a few drinks.)* I knew you wouldn't dig it. You've never lived on the edge . . . try to see hell, touch the sky.

GAF: Living on the edge of physical experience?

Jim: That's where it is, man, everything else is illusion, boring. Danger is real. Death is the ultimate gig.

GAF: Does this view of life affect your work? *(I am unfamiliar with the Doors.)*

Jim: Of course. We're sexual politicians. We get people off, move them over the edge into orgasm. If you're Freudian you must have read Norman Brown—you know about man's repression by society. *(Smiles broadly)* I'm kind of like you . . a healer, a shaman, treating the fucked up, the repressed. But I use music and poetry to help to liberate people. I'm able to free them from their neuroses, get them beyond the blinders and the rules. I excite them, arouse their anger and pain . . . their sexuality, to get to their impulses. *(Jim is becoming more verbal, but his manner is still bland and low key.)*

GAF: *(I remain silent while Jim is beginning to become a bit relaxed and expansive. Perhaps he is taking the opportunity to espouse his views. Still, at times he seems distracted. There is a slight smirk on his face as he speaks.)*

Jim: Of course, the judge and the cops and the lawyers are just as fucked up as everybody else, they just don't know it. I want every experience to try and go beyond the ordinary . . . the rules . . . the limits imposed by society. You can't get anywhere until you get past the shit and sharpen your senses . . . to touch the boundaries of existence. Even death, it's the ultimate experience and I don't want to go out unconscious and miss it. *(A brief silence)* Jimi Hendricks and Janis have already checked out but the word is that they were high. Not me, I won't be. Death is a door, something to go through and be transformed, like the shaman . . . . *(After a pause, he shifts emotionally, as if in slow motion.)* Have you read Rimbaud or Blake or Poe or Kafka? They understood.

GAF: How long have you been thinking about checking out?

Jim: Always. The final boundary. People are afraid, they don't understand that death is freedom. You don't understand either, do you? *(Condescending, Jim is now warming up a bit and appears slightly more alert.)* It's too bad, you should understand. Freud had a bit of it . . . a glimmer. He knew that civilized man has been deprived of his impulses and senses . . . that . . . that all real experience, all of man's instincts and drives have been encased in the cement of culture and society. That the raw experience of life is stifled, smothered in rules, commandments, in the demand for order. The only way is back to the subconscious, by becoming aware of all that has been pushed out of our immediate consciousness by civilization. And I know there is one way to get there — by breaking the hold reality has on us, by experiencing everything, breaking through to disorder and the primacy of the senses. Rimbaud knew — sanity through insanity. Blake knew — the doors between the known and the unknown. *(Jim's superior intelligence is obvious and he is now showing an impressive grasp of certain philosophical and psychological ideas, such as the question Freud raised about civilization being the cause of neurotic conflict in man, i.e. civilization fosters the rules that repress most of man's natural instincts. But Jim distorts these ideas to justify his behavior, which is really the result of his struggle with the dead zone.)*

GAF: Are you saying that you get drunk to experience life more fully? Seems to me that being drunk is more like a barrier to fully experiencing anything. Alcohol doesn't expand the senses, it clouds them. *(I've decided to challenge him and create just a little cognitive dissonance around his intellectualizing.)*

Jim: No. No. *(Jim reacts to my challenge. Energized, he sits up and leans forward to engage me more fully. He obviously wants to explain himself now.*) Everything I do is to free me up. I want to experience everything more vividly, more intensely. Huxley used mescaline to expand his consciousness. I want to know things one can't know without changing the way our senses work — to experience the unknown, to find what's meaningful. I've always thought about it. Alcohol is just a part of the trip, and part of stirring things up.

GAF: Could there be other reasons for your search for meaning and experience?

Jim: What do you mean? *(His voice indicating he's becoming annoyed at my probing question)*

GAF: Well, what are existence and experience like for you without expanding the senses?

Jim: Painful . . . death is . . . really a friend because life is pain. Like standing on the down slope of some dark, angry void. *(He is staring slightly now. I'm trying to evaluate his state of mind.)*

GAF: Dark, angry void?

Jim: Yeah . .(*He shifts mood again and becomes hostile, and his narcissism also appears more blatantly.*) What's the matter, can't Freud explain someone like me, or am I just too much for *you*?

GAF: (*Although I cannot know at this point what is going on with Jim, I would tend to address his hostility. And the phrase angry void catches my attention. It may be the poetic language of an intellectual who is depressed, or the words of a cynic. Or maybe neither.*) Maybe you're concerned that I won't be able to explain you? (*I believe he means help him.*) And maybe that scares you and makes you angry? That there may be no help for the pain?

Jim: (*First he looks away angry and disgusted. Then he leans forward and glares at me.*) What a fucking asshole. You don't jerk off enough. You need to get rid of the bullshit and get more pussy. Your mind is dead from too much Freud and too little action. Get fucked. (*Jim's mini-tirade is somewhat moderated by his uncertainty regarding what happens in a therapy session, and by his probation. But I touched a nerve, one very close to his despair.*)

GAF: (*I give him a questioning look, meant to*

ask non-verbally, "what was that all about?". My expectation is that he will be forthcoming once he sees that I'm not intimidated or made angry by his tirade.) What just happened?

Jim: You pissed me off. You think you know something. But you don't. You're just playing shrink games. *(Jim is slowly becoming less agitated and seems to settle back a bit in the chair.)*

GAF: Mmm. You thought my question was part of a game?

Jim: Look, I told you all this doesn't matter. I'm only here because of that cretin of a judge. *(Now sullen)*

GAF: Well, this form of therapy is non-coercive, and the patient comes to explore what things mean to him, why he is self-defeating or what his conflicts are all about—why he is anxious or depressed or angry. They are motivated by the desire to understand. People come to lower their misery level. *(I attempt a little educating here.)*

Jim: You and I are in different worlds. You think everybody's neurotic, and you try to analyze them. I see everybody as fucked. Fucked by all the bullshit that I try to break down. So . . . we have nothing in common. You don't get it. You don't understand! *(Angrily shaking his head)*

GAF: *(I am looking to capture his interest by touching on his emotional stress and intellectual arrogance.)* I understand anguish,   anxiety,   pain, hopelessness, despair.   Maybe there's more to your search than you realize.

Jim: What the fuck are you talking about?

GAF: You mentioned that life is pain, a 'dark angry void.' Is that how it is for you personally? Or was that a rhetorical— *(He cuts me off)*

Jim: So!   That's just the way life is. *(Annoyed and dismissive)*

GAF: *(Trying again)* For you too?

Jim: For everybody. Only some don't know it, they're too numb to it and only know the rules.   *(Appears disgusted)*

GAF: Well. How is it for you to feel that angry void?

Jim: *(Thinking for a moment, he seems to find the question interesting.)* I use it.

I make it work for me, and people use me to come alive instead of staying repressed and bored. *(Jim is slowly being drawn into a philosophical discussion, but his inner feelings are there behind the words.)*

GAF: So you make them feel alive. Just how do you do that?

Jim: By working on them, teasing, taunting . . . and then the music pulls them over the edge and they lose it . . I know just how to do it, to tease it out. *(He's appears proud of his philosophy here, but I find his pose nonetheless unconvincing, leaving me with the impression that he doesn't really believe it.)*

GAF: So you're not feeling repressed and bored when you're doing that for them?

Jim: *(Shakes head)* That's right. It's like magic. Like the shaman who channels everything through himself and takes on their evil impulses and anger. *(Here maybe is a touch of the Christian belief about Christ taking on the sins of man — perhaps a bit of Jim's mysticism and grandiosity.)*

GAF: How are you feeling when you're not taking on the impulses and anger of others? Are you feeling the way they do?

Jim: Yeah. I know how they feel and they know I do, so they respond to me.

GAF: So you know how they feel. You have the same angry void they do. What is it really like for you?

Jim: *(He is angry again. My question challenges his attempts to maintain an intellectual/mystical aura around his feelings so as to keep them controlled. Jim is very smart and isn't going to be easily led to talk about himself at this level.)* Are we finished for today? This is going nowhere. It's pathetic that you sit there thinking you can understand me when you're stuck with this crap job and play these games. You're blind and don't know it. *(Agitated, he turns away from me in his chair, a deep frown on his face.)*

GAF: Perhaps, but it surprises me that you seem to find my question so problematic. *(I continue here to stay on the subject of his angry feeling. Eventually he might find my question harder to ignore.)*

Jim: *(He reacts coolly and with obvious agitation.)* It's no problem. But we

have no common language. You
won't get it, and I'm in no mood to
try to fill you in. So . . . I have to
go.

GAF: Maybe we can try again next time.
(He leaves without further comment.)

Not an unusual session for this type of patient
who can be sullen, arrogant and intellectual. He
nurses his pain with complex ideas and philosophy.
Because he is so intelligent he can challenge and evade
with perspectives and attitudes that the therapist might
find interesting and therefore distracting.

Jim misses the second session and arrives for the
third ten minutes late, disconnected and aloof.

Session 3.

Jim: I can only stay for ten minutes . . . I
have a rehearsal.

GAF: Well, ten minutes won't be helpful
to you, so we should reschedule.

Jim: Okay. See you later. *(He leaves)*

Session 4.

Jim's oppositional tendencies are pronounced.
He would continue to avoid and evade the sessions
until his probation was over, but the probation officer
pulls him in and he arrives for the next session on time.
He is annoyed and recalcitrant. We spar again, but he
does begin to ease up on his negativity because he is
still feeling the dread of the dead zone.

Jim: That little fuck *(the probation officer)* is a pathetic, mindless robot.

GAF: He hassled you?

Jim: Yeah. Checked up on my schedule and found out I missed a session. Then he did his big man speech about, *(mimics)* 'you have to work with me Jim. We can work this out but you've gotta give me some cooperation.' The little fuck . . .

GAF: Mmmn. Well. Maybe we can use the time. You're a man with some interesting ideas and convictions. *(I'm appealing to his intellectual vanity.)*

Jim: Yeah . . . maybe. Go ahead, ask what you want. *(Jim is less agitated with me than in the first session, at least for now.)*

GAF: It's not what I want, it's what you feel about yourself and your life and how we might together find a new way of looking at things. That's what therapy offers. We can learn something and maybe break through the confusion.

Jim: Yeah? What things? What confusion? I'm not the one who's confused. *(Annoyed, he scowls at me.)*

GAF: I meant the confusion between us. It's unclear to me, for example, just what your feelings about life and death are all about.

Jim: I told you what matters. Pain, sex, experiences and death. *(Impatiently)*

GAF: It would help to know how you've come to this view.

Jim: It's obvious isn't it? Look around at people and how stiff and scared and angry they are. They're all looking for a peak experience, to let loose, and they don't know how.

GAF: How can you be sure that people feel that way?

Jim: I read it in their faces . . . in their uptight faces.

GAF: Is it possible that you feel scared and angry, too, and that when you look at them you see the reflection of your own feelings in their faces? *(I'm confronting him once again, suggesting that Jim could be projecting his own anxieties onto others.)*

185

Jim: What? *(Disdainfully)* You can't use that shrink shit on me. I'm seeking the very things that frighten them—letting go, busting out. I don't project onto them, I entice and instigate. I liberate them. *(Jim is laid back in the chair, becoming calmer as he speaks; he is feeling more sure of himself as he uses his intelligence to hide his demons.)*

GAF: What is it like for you to entice and instigate?

Jim: What do you mean?

GAF: What are you feeling when you entice and instigate . . and liberate them? *(I ask about his intentions here because Jim does not seem to be interested in his audiences merely to promote his career, as someone driven purely by the quest for glory. So I'm hoping to push him to explore his real motives.)*

Jim: *(Ponders the question)* I don't know. It's just the way I am. What difference does it make?

GAF: Well, you know, I was wondering what you might be experiencing when you're performing.

Jim: It's a high, a peak experience. At least it used to be, but it's not like that now.   I think that I'm just getting tired. I'm going to move on, maybe publish more of my poetry. (*Then as an afterthought*) I plan to join Pamela in Paris in a few months.

GAF: You're leaving your band?

Jim: Yeah, after the next tour.

GAF: Do I understand you correctly, that you no longer feel the same satisfaction on stage as you once did?

Jim: Yeah, that's right. (*This is the first time Jim has made a direct comment about his personal feelings rather than an intellectual or philosophical argument.*)

GAF: Could you tell me more about what's changed?

Jim: I don't know, things are just different. It's as if none of it matters anymore. I've got to move on, experience everything and get my thoughts together. Work on my poetry. The poets are the only truly tuned-in people. They move along the fault lines of life, they meet the chaos and pain head on . . (*Jim is rambling a bit – the closest he will get to 'free associating' in therapy.*)

187

GAF: You've mentioned the pain of life a few times now. You experience life as painful?

Jim: Yes . . . so? Doesn't everybody? *(Jim, like others living in the dead zone, can't really describe the experience of the dead zone. He tends to project his anxiety onto the world.)*

GAF: Not the way you describe it. How is it so painful for you?

Jim: *(Stares at me for a while. Jim's anger and hostility of the first session are absent now and he sighs, sits back in a more relaxed fashion, and seems to be pondering my question. For a moment I wonder if he is gaining some interest in the therapy. I am wrong.)* You still haven't figured out what I'm talking about. You're a rather disappointing example of your profession. Are you typical? How could you possibly help anyone? You're not smart enough, and you're not experienced enough. *(Jim is speaking slowly and quietly, and in a scornful voice. My question clearly upset him.)*

GAF: My question angers you?

Jim: You're just another flunky doing what you've been trained to do by an ossified discipline and those who fear their own natural instincts. You try to inhibit those who aren't afraid, who seek the truth . . . the poets, for example. What kind of Freudian are you anyway? What kind of training and education did you have that left you so uncomprehending? I would've expected you to appreciate the need for releasing pent-up impulses. Repressing leaves you soft-headed and frustrated. So, why are you so dense?

GAF: You mentioned Freud several times, and seem to have more than a cursory grasp of his ideas. Are you rejecting his concept that we're all moved more by unconscious motives than conscious ones? After all, repression is a defense based on the idea of the unconscious. Or are you saying your motives aren't mostly unconscious like the rest of us? *(I am directly challenging Jim. I have not been able to move him into examining his behavior or to reflect on his repeated angry or defensive reactions to all questions about his personal feelings. His last reaction seems to have been triggered by my effort to focus him on pain in a more personal way. So the challenge is a bit of a risk but is intended to upset his defensive adjustment of projecting and intellectualizing his painful feelings.)*

Jim: See, you're off course again. I know that everything really important is unconscious. Our motives are unconscious. That's why I've been exploring my unconscious for as long as I can remember. And the unconscious is where you find the chaos, the sensuality, and sexuality—really find the essence of life. No rules, no restrictions, no bullshit. It's being, without inhibiting the senses, the inhibition that makes life painful and death friendly. I'm surprised that you find this so difficult to figure out. I don't think I've misjudged you. You can't get it because you're blinded by the game plan of a society that alienates you from yourself. *(Jim's intelligence once again helps him to avoid the implications of my questioning. Here is a good example of how a strength and intelligence can be used to defend against the emergence of threatening but largely unconscious feelings, e.g. dread and despair.)*

GAF: *(I try again.)* I am still puzzled by your reluctance to discuss the pain you mention at a more personal level, as readily as you do at the

190

level of the group and in society. Especially if you maintain, as you do, that you are in touch with your own unconscious.

Jim: You want to know more about pain? Is the concept of pain so hard to understand? Everybody's in pain.

GAF: Well, pain is a more general word for discomfort of some kind, but it's nonspecific. If you're talking about psychological pain, then there are many possibilities — apprehension, worry, anxiety, dread as one continuum for example. Or sadness, grief, depression, despair as another, or agitation, irritability, anger, rage as a third. These can be part of psychological pain, and I can't figure out from what you've told me whether or not in your case any or all of these are involved.

Jim: What difference does it make? It's all the same thing man, can't you see that? Haven't you read Sartre and the existentialists? It's about alienation and about a kind of nonexistence, of nothingness. No feelings . . . no sensation . . . no meaning, no hope.

GAF: No feeling and no hope. Are those

your feelings, too?

Jim: Yeah, like almost everybody else, except most don't even know that they're alienated from themselves. They blindly accept the repression of society and never get beyond it.

GAF: You see the restrictions of society and its rules as the cause of your feelings of hopelessness. Could there be other causes?

Jim: What do you mean? *(An opening, maybe. Jim might be willing to entertain the idea that some of his pain is independent of society.)*

GAF: Well, we haven't discussed your background. Perhaps some of those feelings stem from early experiences. *(At this point, I have yet to realize that Jim may be living in the dead zone. So I'm looking to explore any childhood precipitants of pain.)*

Jim: What early experiences?

GAF: Any that may have shaped your feelings about life and yourself. Since you're familiar with Freud you know that he felt like Wadsworth, that 'the child is father to the man.' We're all shaped by our history. Your relationship with your parents, for example.

Jim: My parents are dead.

GAF: Oh, then I was given an incorrect
       summary by the probation officer.
       He indicated that your parents live
       in Florida, and that your dad is an
       admiral in the Navy. The officer
       talked to the authorities in Florida
       where you apparently had a run-in
       with the law last year.

Jim: Yeah, that's right. But they're dead
       to me.

GAF: How did you come to feel this
       way?

Jim: They're just not important, that's
       all. Let's just move on . .

This session is illustrative of the difficulties
facing a therapist trying to conduct a session with an
unwilling patient. Jim would present problems for any
therapist. First, he is not interested in therapy. Second
he is unwilling to reflect on his inner world, preferring
instead to project his discomforts onto others. And
third, he is unable to acknowledge his background and
provide the historical context for his character and
behavior.   And finally, he uses his intelligence to
challenge the therapist's sense of competence and to
attack. But despite these problems, the therapist has
one ally—Jim's desire to end his own misery. His
intelligence cannot really compensate for the way his
underlying pathology distorts his view of things. By
bringing the distortions into sharp relief and showing a

willingness to explore nonjudgmentally the meaning of behavior and feelings, the therapist can offer hope to the patient. Jim has stayed in session twice, and the hope is that he is starting to feel the beginnings of trust and to hope for relief from the pain.

Jim comes for the fifth session. He is a few minutes late but exhibits none of the arrogant, oppositional behavior of the other sessions. Instead he is milder in manner and even looks a bit depressed. He looks at me expectantly.

Session 5.

Jim: *Jim is dressed in black, looking very tired, almost defeated.*)   So what do we talk about today?

GAF: Well, how have things gone for you this week?

Jim: I don't know. I'm just tired of it all. Nothing feels good. So what do you make of that? *(Jim may be feeling the chaos and emptiness of the dead zone now. Perhaps he's hoping I can help somehow, yet at the same time he feels the despair that is always with him.   But at this point, I cannot diagnose the cause of his despair.)*

GAF: It makes me wonder about what could be going on. In spite of your success, you   feel   tired   and dissatisfied.

Jim: *(He looks at me, apparently trying to decide   whether   to   respond   to   my*

194

comment or to ignore it. He sits silently for a few moments and then with a look that appears to be a mixture of anticipation and disdain, he seems ready to put down whatever I say. Yet part of him is still hopeful.) Yeah, well, you're the shrink. What do your books say?

GAF: Sometimes 'feeling tired' and 'nothing feeling good' are symptoms of depression. Sometimes they are symptoms of an internal conflict as in Pogo's famous line "we have met the enemy and he is us." We need a little more detail about these symptoms before we can make sense of them.

Jim: Detail? Like what? *(Jim is reluctantly drawn in by what is left of hope in him. But that hope is just a distant flicker of light.)*

GAF: Like how you feel in different settings, how you feel about your work, how you act in intimate relationships. Freud, when asked about what constituted emotional health, supposedly said the ability "to love and to work." Are you able to love and to work, and to be gratified?

Jim: Huh! You mean fuck and write?

Yeah. So?

GAF: Maybe there's more to it. Fucking is not loving. And you say that you're not feeling very good, that you feel miserable. Can you elaborate?

Jim: Elaborate what? I'm tired and fed up. The whole scene has become boring and meaningless. I need to get away, work on my poetry. *(Jim trails off. After a few moments he returns to his lament, in a vague, mournful voice.)* I don't feel the excitement anymore. The whole thing is . . . irrelevant. I . . . need to find . . . I don't know what I want to do. Don't even know who I am, what I want. Have you ever read Camus' novel *The Stranger*? I know that guy, I know where he's coming from. Problem is, he's all fucked up. *(I found this to be a remarkable admission from Jim, considering his sulk in previous sessions. He stares out the window.)*

GAF: *(I am alerted by this last comment about The Stranger. The character in Camus' book is a good example of someone living in the dead zone.)* That guy is detached and alienated from himself and from life. Is that how you feel?

196

Jim: That's right. He can't get into it. There's nothing there or anywhere that makes any difference to him. He doesn't really experience anything. All he does is tolerate the bullshit. So he has no hope.

GAF: You're feeling hopeless then?

Jim: You could say that. *(Still in a contemplative mood.)* What would justify hope? Nothing in life is hopeful because the meaning of existence is hidden behind the conventions of civilization. *(Jim falls into his intellectual defenses now.)* Action's better than inaction, chaos is better than order, sex is better than chastity, death is better than life. I've told you all this. Only people who don't comprehend this can fool themselves into being hopeful.

GAF: *(Challenging Jim directly here would only harden his defenses. Instead, I try to increase trust and form an alliance with Jim by staying focused on his subjective experience of himself and life. So I will ask him how he feels about the way he feels.)* It must be very hard to walk around without hope. How is it for you to feel the way you do?

Jim: *(Jim readily understands this question. He looks up and becomes more intense as he describes himself.)* It gives me a sense of power. I'm not stopped by common fears. Having no belief in the ordinary, I can take on anything, challenge all the petty bullshit, live on the edge, closer to the boundary between smothering social mores and the liberating qualities of sex, drugs, and death. Christ had a piece of it. Lose yourself to find yourself.

GAF: Uh huh. You've resigned yourself to hopelessness and find yourself free to defy the world. You have no fear because you have no hope.

Jim: That's right . . you're finally getting it. *(But Jim does not strike me as feeling good about his success in helping me to "finally get it." He looks tormented still.)*

GAF: What if you're wrong?

Jim: What are you talking about?

GAF: What if your conclusions about why you feel hopeless are wrong? What if the reasons for your agitation and despair are not what you believe them to be?

Jim: Yeah . . . okay . . . What's your theory? *Jim's voice signals to me that while he doesn't dare let hope enter into his life, he does hope.)*

GAF: *(I will try to capture his interest again as he seems ready to consider alternatives to his views. I am now aware that he may be living in the dead zone. I will try to use Camus' The Stranger to make it easier for Jim to consider that he may also feel the dead zone.)* You say you feel like the stranger? From my point of view, the stranger was alienated from himself and all others as well. He was living with an existential despair that was always part of him, a sense of nothingness that did not derive from the suppression of his instincts and senses, but from unknown developmental glitches in his identity formation and in his ability to attach to others. He would have felt this way as long as he could recall– questioning reality, seeking to be aroused or excited in order to escape the nothingness, or to quiet the dread and agitation that are part of the despair. Is that true for you? That you've always felt this way? *(I'm checking a hypothesis by using Camus' character.)*

Jim: Yeah . .

GAF: And you find that excitement changes your experience of the nothingness?

Jim: Yeah, maybe.

GAF: Could it be that your insistence on action, sensation, sex, and intense experiences are your way of gaining relief from the nothingness and the inner agitation?

Jim: *(Jim reflects on these ideas, and his intelligence helps him here. But at the same time he is oppositional, narcissistic, and hostile, therefore unpredictable. But now he is quiet.)* Maybe . . maybe.

GAF: If you recall, *The Stranger* was unmoved by the death of his mother. Even committing murder left him without feeling of any kind.   So intense experiences didn't help him. Do I understand you correctly, that you might be feeling that way?

Jim: Yeah . . . maybe.   Not a bad theory, but . . *(Jim remains attentive, pensive and slightly skeptical. But he is still listening.)*

GAF: Have you felt this way, this

nothingness, as long as you can remember?

Jim: Yeah. *(Jim's looking more despondent as we talk. Then, after some time passes, Jim looks at me expectantly.)* So what about it? Your theory's not bad. But it's not new. I've known that all along. What difference does it make? You're talking about a kind of, uh, developmental glitch? *(Notice how Jim has just accepted an alternative way of explaining his troubles by appropriating it as his own and as not new. His challenge to me, "What difference does it make?" is offered in the hope that I might be able to help without him asking for it.)*

GAF: Well, maybe we can explore it together, maybe find ways to ease up the agitation and soften the nothingness. We might find some answers for the alienation. It depends on understanding your experiences better than we do.

Jim: Yeah . . . understanding what?

GAF: Well, for example, can you get hold of your inner state of feeling when you are not performing, not drinking, and not taking drugs? Can you describe what it's like to be you under ordinary

201

circumstances?

Jim: I don't know, maybe. It's just like the way things are, like boring, meaningless. *(long silence)* I don't know.

GAF: Boring and agitating at the same time?

Jim: Yeah. And unreal. *(Here again is the dead zone paradox. The person is feeling empty and emotionally turbulent at the same time, i.e., bored and agitated.)*

GAF: Unreal?

Jim: Yeah . . . unreal. You know, like when you feel as if, as though you're a mechanical man, or maybe like you're acting in a play and not really there. As though everything was a dream, like you were ethereal . . . amorphous . . . like you're just a two-dimensional profile, without any substance or reality. Rimbaud . . . uhhhh. So . . *(drifts off)* It's what I've been telling you — everything is so goddamned controlled and orderly that you can't feel anything. Your senses are atrophied, no experience of excitement, of reality. It's all the same problem. Civilization destroys the real meaning of things.

GAF: I don't think that's sufficient to explain your feelings.

Jim: What do you mean?

GAF: I don't think that civilization, or the law, or the rules of society have anything to do with what you're experiencing. I've seen people who feel the way you do, and they all attempt to figure out why. Each has some explanation, as you do. But it seems to be that each has feelings similar to you and to the character in Camus' novel, and those feelings. . . of existential despair are not the result of social forces in my experience.

Jim: So what are you saying, that there's something wrong with me? *(Jim is alert in the face of my confrontation, but there is still a bland, intellectualized quality to his questioning of me.)*

GAF: I'm saying that we need to look inside you for the answers to your feeling of boredom and agitation.

Jim: Yeah? Interesting idea. How's that any different than what I've been doing? Living on the edge, experiencing everything, no limits? I'm trying to experience the inside. *(drifting off)*

GAF: My impression is that you've been escaping from the feelings, not exploring them. Experiencing the outer world isn't the same as reflecting on the inner one. And as a good example, as I mentioned earlier, it would be helpful to know what you're feeling when just being quiet and alone. You said 'bored and unreal.' How is that for you? What's it like?

Jim: *(Jim looks at me and shrugs. For a moment there is a far away look, a sense of preoccupation quickly followed by a return to a matter-of-fact attitude. Jim has gone as far as he can today.)* I don't know. It's just there. I've got another recording session today. Have to go . .

GAF: Okay.

Jim came close to touching the dread within. But he is caught in the dilemma of having defended against it by rationalizing it as a by-product of society's conventions and therefore something to be "broken through" rather than resolved by self-reflection. He returns for the next session on time. He is subdued, non-combative and non-responsive. The likely explanation is that he felt some part of the dead zone and some sense of being understood, which both attracts and repels him at the same time.

Session 6.

Jim: *(Again he's dressed in black as seems to befit his mood. Avoiding eye contact, perhaps to avoid being upset like the last time, he slowly sits down, blanking starring at me, saying nothing.)*

GAF: How are things?

Jim: Fine.

GAF: Have you had any thoughts about our last session?

Jim: No.

GAF: Mmm. I'm surprised at that. We seemed to have found some common ground. I wonder how you felt when you left?

Jim: Fine.

GAF: Mmm, well I ask because it seemed to me that we were beginning to sort some things out and that at the end of the session you felt better understood. Is that correct, or did I misread you?

Jim: Yeah, it was okay. So . . . now what? What am I supposed to do now? What difference does it all make? *(Jim is calm and detached. Part of him has withdrawn from the threat of being understood as he was in the previous session, while another part of him desperately wants to connect.)*

GAF: Well that depends on what you want.   If you're interested in working on the nothingness and the alienation . . . if you don't want to feel like Camus' stranger, then there are some things we can do. But it'll take time and work.

Jim: *(Looks down and away as if considering my comments.)* How do we do that? Don't tell me this is all about Freud and the Oedipus complex.

GAF: Not quite.   It's not about the Oedipus complex.   *(In fact, Jim would be better off if it were. But his difficulties are based on disturbances that develop prior to the age at which Oedipal conflicts tend to emerge-ages 3 to 5.)* Feelings of nothingness and unreality are outcomes that tend to originate before Oedipal conflicts develop. Say before age 2 ½ to 3.

Jim: Before? You mean before 3? *(Jim appears genuinely surprised.)*

GAF: Yes, but the developmental glitch

affects   all   subsequent developmental stages as well.

Jim: What can go wrong before the age of three? Christ!

GAF: We don't really know the cause, only the consequences.

Jim: *(Again looking off, out the window at trees bared of their leaves in the cold November light. He looks anguished to the depths of his being and one guesses that Jim is ever so lightly touching on his deepest despair.)* Look at that *(he points to the outside.)* It's sterile—no life, no sensation, no existence. Nothing tangible . . . like me. *(almost to himself and sounding exhausted.)* Ohhh . . . God!

GAF: *(I can feel Jim's torment and I become more certain that he is living in the dead zone.)* You're living in dread of this nothingness, trying to find meaning in it. Perhaps it's time to contend with it.

Jim: Yeah? Maybe. How?   If you're right and it started that fucking early, what can I do?   What the fuck can I do? It's not like there's a drug I can take. I already do that. Even Freud can't fix this. *(Jim is verbally negative but hoping that he is wrong about Freud, and that I really can help him.)*

GAF: Well, the more we understand your experience the better we can help you organize it, reduce it, contain it, and then integrate it with the rest of your personality. I know all these psychoanalytic ideas are complex and abstract. But they're powerfully explanatory. They enable us to help you work through your experience of nothingness and unreality.

Jim: Why nothingness? Why's everything unreal? *(Jim is very smart and thus having some way to comprehend his dilemma may be a critical need. Many patients do not want or need as much understanding as he might.)*

GAF: There are some excellent concepts that seem to account for these things. We can discuss them along the way if you wish. They wouldn't be very helpful to you right now.

Jim: Yeah? Well how much time will it take? *(Now Jim returns to a more guarded place—mistrust is a byproduct of living in the dead zone. There is neither relief nor a moment when the deadness isn't felt. In the face of that kind of immutability, who there could imagine trusting that it can change?)*

GAF: That's uncertain. It's a very complicated problem and it may be several years.

Jim: Several years! Several years!

GAF: Well, you've lived with it all your life. It'll take a while to resolve it.

Jim: I don't get it yet. What happens before three? What could have happened to account for this? How do you know? *(His intelligence requires some cognitive grasp of the these possibilities. He again raises the question and grapples with it, a sign at times of hopefulness in the patient.)*

GAF: It's not easy to understand. We don't really know. There are many possibilities. The best clinical minds have attempted to explain, for example, your persistent conflict in relationships, your constant seeking of excitement, your tendency to withdraw, the contradictions, the impulsiveness, and the acting out behaviors as defenses against feelings of aloneness and high anxiety in infancy and early childhood — whatever the source of the anxiety.

The nothingness, the sense of unrealness, and the despair can be seen as the result of the continued use of these defenses. To be sure, the defenses are very primitive. This is because they're developed early in life and never evolve into more advanced forms.

Jim: Defenses? How can feeling nothing and unreal be defenses? Didn't Freud . . . aren't defenses supposed to help? *(Again, Jim's intellect is at work here. He's asking rather sophisticated questions.)*

GAF: Yes, but the feelings of nothingness and unreality are not the defenses. They're the by-product stemming from the continued use of the only defenses available at those ages, that is— agitation, fantasy-formation, withdrawal from attachment, motoric action, and the separation of all experiences into good and bad feelings and images. And there is a mental process called splitting. Using the only defenses available to an infant and not having them evolve as the child grows can result in the feelings of dread, despair, emotional unevenness, and a special kind of inner aloneness.

Jim: Yeah? So you think you have the answers to this shit? How can you be sure? What evidence do you have? *(Jim is intrigued by the discussion, but his fundamental reason for asking these questions is, again, to elicit some possibility of hope.)*

GAF: Jim, the questions you ask have been and continue to be addressed in the clinical literature. I wonder if . . . if you're having difficulty holding back your doubt and mistrust because following rules and, uh . . customs or the social conventions have never relieved those feelings of dread and agitation before.

Jim: *(Jim is reflecting on my comments and stares off again.)* Nothing changes the way it is, or relieves it. Of course I doubt it. My experiences have taught me . . . that there's no means of escape from the numbing of . . . civilization. You argue from . . . within that perspective. You're without experience in my world of expanded awareness . . . and without the openness to consider it. You're smarter than I first gave you credit for. You've made a few good points, but I can't see that you're going to make any real difference. *(Jim is scared and confused, but he cannot let himself* *trust or hope because he has a low tolerance for disappointment or frustration. It is threatening to him and so he cannot risk it – another by-product of the dead zone. Yet he is desperate about his inner chaos and he is now challenging me to convince him there is hope.)*

GAF: You're right, I haven't experienced the nothingness and the unreality that you talk about. But I am familiar with those experiences clinically. In fact, almost everyone has had a few seconds, here and there, when a sense of nothingness and unreality happen. But it's too fleeting to cause the trouble you're having. And frankly, I doubt that assigning the blame for your feelings to civilization will help. It really hasn't helped, has it?

Jim: *(Smiling wryly. He is taking the challenge well, but he cannot accept my comments without diminishing them somehow.)* You have Freud's work to help support your position, and that's cool. But Freud knew that people were all fucked up by the rules and the bullshit, by civilization's contradictions. How can you ignore that part of Freud? You must have read Norman Brown.

GAF: I hope we find that your take on the cause of your struggle is wrong.

Jim: What? Why?

GAF: Well, if civilization is the problem, it's difficult to see how civilization can change enough in our lifetime to help with the despair you feel. *(I'm falling down here. It will not help Jim if I am drawn into a theoretical discussion. What he is again asking indirectly, is, "Can you really help?")*

Jim: Yeah? What if you're right?

GAF: I don't see the problem that way. It seems that what we need is a way of understanding what you're experiencing and some way of working through the despair.

Jim: Yeah. I don't know. Maybe. What do we do?

GAF: Next time we meet I'll outline the way to proceed, if you choose to continue.

Jim: Yeah, okay.

Jim has come around a bit and we might be able to initiate psychotherapy. It remains to be seen whether he will really invest in the work. His need-fear dilemma is apparent. He desperately seeks relief from the constant emotional tumult, yet feels threatened by any chance of a connection to others. He will be unwavering in his detachment. His next appointment is canceled by his office. He shows up the following week for the eighth session. He has now come for two sessions more than required by the judge.

Session 8.

GAF: Good afternoon.

Jim: Hi.

GAF: Have you thought any further about the last session?

Jim: Yeah, some. Guess I'll see how it goes for a while.

GAF: *(This is the time to advise Jim on the basics for this form of therapy.)* Okay, let's discuss the way this form of therapy works and the basic requirements for it to work, to see if we can agree on a sort of contract. My responsibility will be to provide you with three weekly sessions at fixed times. The sessions will last fifty minutes. My commitment is to listen carefully and try to understand what you're experiencing. When I have an observation or comment to offer, I will. Your part will be to talk about yourself, your background, and current difficulties. If there are no specific problems at the time, then you should talk about any thoughts, feelings, behaviors, memories, dreams and perceptions that come to mind. The more freely you communicate what's on your mind, the more we can learn, because in that way the significant conflicts and concerns usually surface. In a sense, it's the psychological equivalent of 'all roads lead to Rome.' Even if what passes through your mind at times seems inconsequential, it may assist us at some point if you verbalize it. My helpfulness to you depends on your efforts to make clear what you do know about yourself. At times, your thinking about these things will cause you to ask questions. I may not always answer, depending on my assessment of what would be most helpful to you at that time. Thus communications in therapy are a bit different than in ordinary conversation. How does this description feel to you so far? *(This contract or explicit agreement on the specifics of the process is essential if we are to avoid the diversions and distractions that would be brought by the chaos of the borderline's inner world. The compact is to be used, in concert with psychoanalytic concepts regarding this complicated condition, to stay on course and keep the patient and therapist focused on the patient's internal state. It also reassures the patient about the steadfastness of the therapist and the predictability of the process. Thus, it goes a long way toward giving the patient the only sense of object constancy he may have ever experienced.)*

Jim: Yeah. Okay. What about gigs and tours out of state?

GAF: Well, those things can't be helped. We'll have to work around them as best we can.

Jim: And I have a problem with several years. I don't know where I'll be in a year.

GAF: Yes, those are concerns, but we'll have to deal with them one at a time if you decide to proceed. It's very important that we both understand and agree on the framework for this form of therapy. Do you have any other questions or comments?

Jim: No, that's cool. But I don't see where this is going.

GAF: We'll have to let it unfold, create a

narration, a construction of sorts that clarifies and reveals. *(I'm being deliberately abstract here, yet Jim may be intrigued.)*

Jim: All right, how do we begin? *(Slouched comfortably in his chair.)*

GAF: So you find the framework acceptable? No concerns?

Jim: Yeah ..

GAF: Well, we've already begun in a way. Talk about whatever comes to mind, as you have been doing.

Jim: I'm still not sure about you.

GAF: How do you mean?

Jim: You seem too formal, stiff . . . too rigid.

GAF: How does that cause you difficulty?

Jim: I can't talk to a stiff. You won't get it.

GAF: Won't get it?

Jim: Yeah.

GAF: I'm not following you.

Jim: Your obsolete thinking and ideas will get in the way of understanding what I'm saying.

GAF: You mean I can't allow for your points of view because my training and experience are —

Jim: You may want to understand, but you really can't. Maybe you could get just a little of it, but not most of what my experience is all about.

GAF: And holding to my narrow views means I can't connect with your experiences in anyway useful to you?

Jim: You have your ideas and they might be useful to some.

GAF: In what way?

Jim: Who knows? *(Jim is now back to oppositional, mistrustful behavior — as I expected he would be.)*

GAF: So you'd really be wasting your time because my thinking is obsolete?

Jim: Yeah . . . it . . . it's uh, possible you have something of a spirit, a feeling for more than this. *(indicating the office and the 'civilized' world. Another part of Jim is hoping he's wrong and that I can get it and help him.)* But you're limited by your obsolete thinking.

GAF: So your sense of me is that I can't be of help to you because I don't have the right perspective. How would you feel different if I had the right one?

Jim: Maybe I could see some point to continuing this.

GAF: You've changed your mind then?

Jim: Changed my mind?

GAF: Yes. In our last session you seemed to think that we might do some exploring together. Now you're saying you don't think we can. How do you account for the change? *(Jim experienced me as positive and helpful in the last session, but it appears he now experiences me as useless: an ever-shifting dichotomy of polarized characteristics, in this instance helpful-vs-useless. So I am clarifying and confronting this shift in his internal experiences. These shifts in his attitude toward the external world are a constant source of confusion and disruption in his personal relationships.)*

Jim: Well, I . . . *(He shrugs and turns*

away, a look of sadness on his face.)

GAF: You know, I have a sense of something from you that I'll pass on if you wish.

Jim: Yeah?

GAF: I noticed during each of the sessions, that you seem to be on guard, apparently scrutinizing me, without revealing very much in the way of facial expression. You appear very controlled. Sometimes you seem detached, as if you feel antagonistic, skeptical that I might be, uh, an adversary in some way, and that you need to remain cool and defiant.

Jim: Yeah . . . probably.

GAF: As if I were an inquisitor.

Jim: *(He shrugs again.)*

GAF: So perhaps your change of attitude is connected with this other view you have of me as a kind of antagonist, an enemy, and you resist reasoning that I have anything to offer you after all.

Jim: Yeah? Maybe. So what?

GAF: So . . . maybe you're expecting also

that I have the same feeling of hopelessness that you do. Surely I couldn't help you in that case. On the other hand, you have engaged in discussion with me, have heard some of my thoughts. You've also showed up for two more sessions than required, and agreed to the idea of exploring your life further with me via the framework we discussed last time.

Jim: So what? (*Eyebrows raised and lips curled up on one side.*)

GAF: Well, it seems to me that you're contending with powerful, malevolent unconscious forces that cause you to experience me as an antagonist who's powerless because of the very fact that I'm trying to help. And you then begin to think of me as being antagonistic toward you while believing you to be hopeless.

Jim: That's really stretching . . .

GAF: Perhaps my observation is off the mark.

Jim: I didn't say you were antagonistic.

GAF: Mmm. Someone to be opposed?

Jim: No, not necessarily. I don't think

your conclusions are valid. *(Jim withdraws into a long silence.)*

GAF: You appear to be reflecting on something. Remember how this therapy works. You should relate what's on your mind to me in as unconstrained a manner as you can. Are you unable to talk about it?

Jim: No. I just want to know what's next.

GAF: I've reviewed with you how we must proceed. We're supposed to be exploring whatever's on your mind.

Jim: But I still don't feel that you can understand.

GAF: So my observation didn't help you to see how it is that you experience me that way?

Jim: I guess not.

GAF Well then, what do you think?

Jim: *(Stares off for a while.)* I don't know . . . I don't feel anything about it one way or the other.

GAF: But the result is you're not going to engage the process of therapy —

not going to talk?

Jim: I guess not.

GAF: Something in you is telling you to keep quiet?

Jim: Yeah, I suppose.

GAF: Your reluctance to speak and acknowledging that seems to validate my observation, wouldn't you say?

Jim: What do you mean?

GAF: You see in me something you're unable to see in yourself— antagonism and hopelessness. Yet it's the malevolent element within you that's in charge, urging you to be uncooperative with the process. To be uninvested, bland, cool. Don't trust . . . keep him on the hook.

Jim: Why should I if I don't think you or anyone can help?

GAF: That would seem b be specious reasoning. If you believe nothing and no one can help, why not just give up and end it. Your intelligence is being used here to support the malevolent elements within.

Jim: Yeah . .

GAF: Hmm.   We seem to have come
       upon a critical piece of your
       conflict—the siren call of relief,
       coming from a part of you that
       urges you to resist, to oppose and,
       if necessary, die. We've found the
       enemy and he is you. You might
       even attempt suicide tonight to
       underscore your resistance and
       hopelessness.

Jim: Yeah . . . so what?

GAF: You make my case.

Jim: Huh?

GAF: You're destroying the therapy by
       remaining silent and by wasting
       our time together, in part because
       you see me as the one who is
       antagonistic and as unable to help.

Jim: *(Silence. The session ends.)*

   By carefully examining the nature of the
interaction in the session, I am trying to make the point
that what happens in the therapy hour is as significant
as what happens outside.   During this last session, I
was attempting to clarify the hidden forces of his inner
world that he projects onto me. I therefore describe the
emotional tone of the hour to him, point out the roles
he has created for me and himself, and identify the

play he is enacting with me. I am attempting to demonstrate how he externalizes a part of the dramatic conflict going on in his internal, psychological world.

Jim arrives for his next session still in his doubting mood but slightly more active.

Session 9.

Jim: What do we do today?

GAF: Talk about whatever comes to mind.

Jim: Yeah, what difference does it make to you? I mean, you sound pretty sure of yourself. What makes you interested in doing this?

GAF: I'm interested, but you'll just have to accept that up front. The real question is how we can overcome the part of you that will readily sabotage our work together. *(This problem of self-sabotage will remain throughout the whole of the therapeutic process.)*

Jim: Why bother then, if that's the case?

GAF: Well, there's another side of you that wants to work, wants to live and get healthier. You've returned, you're asking questions, and you haven't acted to do harm to yourself—as if one part of you is hopeful and votes yes for living

225

and the other is hopeless and votes no. The latter part can't stop thinking of me as hopeless and as a threat even as we talk.

Jim: Maybe. I still don't think you can understand.

GAF: Again, your saying that reflects one of the ways you use your intelligence to rationalize, end treatment, and eventually end your life.

Jim: Yeah . . Well, what now?

GAF: What comes to mind? As we discussed. *(Repetition is to be constant.)*

Jim: *(Silence. Jim looks calmly and blankly at me.)* Not much.

GAF: That's unlikely. It's hard to avoid having something on one's mind for very long. I also get the impression that you remain cynical about our work from the hint of a smirk on your face. So I must assume that you do not take our agreement very seriously and you're not saying what's on your mind. If so, we have to examine the reasons for your silence. One possible reason for your hesitancy is that you feel apprehensive or fearful of revealing yourself. But you don't appear as though you're fearful. Another possibility, based on our previous discussion, is that once again you're kept in a stalemate by the internal conflict between the part of you that seeks relief and the other part that seeks death. The healthy side is what gets you to the therapy sessions and on time, though it's no longer required. Yet the other side seems determined to frustrate us, and I see your passivity and silence as your giving in to that part.

Jim: What of it? What can be done?

GAF: What do *you* want to do?

Jim: So you're going to play Freud and not answer any questions? I ask and you won't answer?

GAF: Well, let me remind you of the way this therapy works.

Jim: So I can't ask questions. You and Freud dictate. *(Defiantly looking around my office, Jim has noticed the psychoanalytic literature on my shelves and, of course, will use it to justify continuing his conflict with the therapy and himself.)*

GAF: You may ask. I'll answer some

and not others, as I outlined to you in earlier sessions.

Jim: But I'm asking you a direct question. Are you going to simply ignore it, and act as though you didn't hear it? Is that what you call therapeutic? Or are you just mimicking Freud like a good little disciple?

GAF: Okay. Perhaps I should help you recall our earlier discussion about the way we must agree to work in this form of therapy. It requires that you say whatever comes to mind without filtering it and that I offer my thoughts when they seem worthwhile. If your thoughts sometimes result in a question, I may answer or I may not, depending on my judgment as to whether a response might benefit you.

Jim: So, if you feel like it, right? Rather capricious of you, isn't it?

GAF: No, I'll respond if I feel it's helpful to you.

Jim: Yeah. So, Dr. Freud, you want to know about my life, all the gory details? *(Jim is not really giving up, but rather is just taking a new approach, although the part of him that seeks health is also present at the very moment that he is being difficult.)* You want to know about my friends?

GAF: Friends?

Jim: Yeah, like Pam, or Ray and Bobby and John?

GAF: Pam, Ray, Bobby, John?

Jim: Pam, my girl. She's cool. We fight . . . and make up. Ray, Bobby and John—my friends. You know I met Janis Joplin a while ago. She was a tough chick. It's too bad . . . about her death, I mean. We met at a party. She's a crazy bitch, whacked me in the head with a bottle. But I still think she was terrific.

GAF: You and Pam live together?

Jim: Yeah, couple of years now. (*Again slouched in his chair.*)

GAF: How is that relationship going?

Jim: You know. It's a relationship, uhh, with no rules, no restrictions. But she's my girl.

GAF: No restrictions?

Jim: Right. We do what feels good.

We're not bound by the limits most people put on each other in relationships. I won't be bound by a straight jacket even if it comes in the form of society's mores. Even if it's accepted by everybody else.

GAF: *(I have a choice here: to address the effect of no rules on the relationship with Pam, or ask for clarification on how he is feeling when he has a need to engage in the extra-relationship activities.)* Do you find that when it's just you and Pam alone for a long time that you get antsy? That you feel the urge to go out and get action, an urge that's separate from your ideas about society's rules?

Jim: Huh . . . no. I see myself as an adventurer, an explorer. I seek meaning . . . meaning. Not walls, not bullshit. *(Jim is speaking, calmly, confidently, but I interpret his response here as a denial of his real inner agitation.)*

GAF: So when you go out to seek adventure, you're engaged in an intellectual and sensory exploration?

Jim: Yeah, that's right. You're thinking that my exploring is really something else?

GAF: Well, I wonder. From a psychoanalytic point of view, of course . . . I wonder if your need for action in this way has other, unconscious motives.

Jim: Yeah? Like what?

GAF: Relief? Distraction? Protection?

Jim: What are you talking about? *(Jim has forgotten our discussion about how he constantly experiences despair.)*

GAF: How is it for you not to go out, to stay with Pam instead?

Jim: It's fine sometimes. But it can get boring. I need to try everything, experience everything. Can't you . . . you must have a dull life if you don't get it, what I'm talking about.

GAF: Boring. You've used that word a lot. *(Boredom is a word used frequently by those in the dead zone when they try to identify their feelings of emptiness.)*

Jim: So? That's the way it is. With dulled senses and no way to bypass society's agenda, everything is boring.

GAF: Boring. Are there other feelings

associated with it?

Jim: I don't know. (*irritated*) Who cares? What the fuck is the matter with you? I'll bet you were a four-eyed twit, teacher's pet, scared of girls and a bore as a kid. What was your class standing? Bottom quarter, right? How can you do this for a living? Can't you get a real job? (*My question may have raised disturbing feelings in Jim, that is, put him in touch with the dread of the dead zone.*)

GAF: (*Brief silence as I let him stay with his hostility a bit.*) You found my question annoying. But our agreement was to explore the nature and meaning of your feelings, ideas, perceptions, behaviors, dreams. Remember?

Jim: Yeah, but that question's stupid. I don't know what you're talking about.

GAF: Mmm. Your angry reaction suggests to me that you do know. If I'm right, we should look to understand why you became so angry and avoided my question.

Jim: (*Silence*) We're finished for today? Isn't time up?

GAF: Yes, see you next time.

Jim: Yeah . . . maybe.

Once again Jim's behavior in this session reveals the difficulty in treating this kind of patient, who often cannot recognize or acknowledge the forces that drive him. Touching on the dead zone elicits feelings of chaos and despair, so Jim attacked me when I pointed that out to him. He seeks relief from these feelings through the use of the defenses of intellectualization, avoidance, and the projection of his malicious dark side onto others. He is truly a man in a titanic struggle for his soul, for his own psychological existence.

Session 10.

Jim returns for a tenth session.

Jim: I'm going on my last tour next week so I won't be here.

GAF: Uh huh. When will you return?

Jim: In about eleven days.

GAF: Is it your intention to continue here?

Jim: Maybe. I guess so. I'll see when I get back.

GAF: Well, we'll have to come to an agreement about your absences. The noncommittal way that you're leaving therapy reduces our

233

chances of successfully treating you and doesn't square with your agreement to operate according to the framework we've agreed on. If you feel you're unable to fulfill your part of the agreement, then we should terminate our work until you feel more ready. *(I am giving Jim reassurance that I will not allow him to undermine the therapy by acquiescing to the forces in him which seek to defeat it.)*

Jim: What, are you kidding? Trying to be a hardass huh? So you won't let me decide when I get back?

GAF: You've already decided. That is, the part of you that kept you coming after your probation was up and the part of you that asked questions and searched for meaning—that part of you did decide. And now, once again, the self-destructive part is here, blocking your momentum toward health by being purposely vague about continuing.

Jim: Jesus! You're blowing this thing up. I have to go on tour. Is that so hard for your little mind to follow? What the fuck do you want—a guarantee written in blood? *(I am not being difficult. Jim can only benefit from this work if he can find a*

*predictability in the therapy and in me.
And the framework for the process and
his collaboration within that framework
can provide the anchor, the constant
reference point for a man who has so
little – almost no identity, tenuous
attachments to others, and numbing
pain about himself and his life.)*

GAF: No, I'm simply reminding you that
this therapy cannot work unless
both of us adhere to the contract.
You'll have to trust my judgment
on this point.

Jim: All right, all right. I'll be here for
the next appointment after I return.
Satisfied? You're making a federal
case out of a simple tour. What're
you going to do when I leave for
France in a few months? My last
concert's in December, the twelfth I
think, and then I'm finished with it
all. Out!

GAF: That'll be your decision. I can
arrange for you to see someone
there, but it'll depend on your
readiness to continue.

Jim: Yeah. Well I'm going. I'm a poet,
that's what I was meant to be. I
had a reading of my poetry last
week. I didn't have time to
mention it last time because you
were busy detailing the therapy.

Poetry's my thing, man, and I intend to be what I should have been all along, a poet. *(Long silence)* Pam's back. She fucked that imbecile Count she knew from Paris. *(Jim appears sad here for just a moment.)* She found me with Patricia. *(Pat Kennealy, an enigmatic, self-proclaimed witch, whom Jim married in an occult ceremony while wearing a black robe, mixing blood, etc. It isn't certain what Jim thought of this marriage.)* She found us bare-assed on the floor . . . She'll get over it. *(Pam Courson had just returned from Paris. From what I could tell, she was the only constant figure in a life consumed by turmoil. This may be part of his reason for returning to her again and again despite their fights and his philosophy of no rules.)*

GAF: Silence.

Jim: Do you read anything but this stuff *(pointing to the books around my office)*, like poetry? Are you familiar with the Greek and Roman mythologies — Dionysus, Apollo? *(Jim looks at me expectantly and after a few moments glares at me.)* What, asking intelligent questions offends your sensibilities? So you're not going to answer any questions?

GAF: As we agreed . . . when I feel it might be useful. *(Before responding to Jim's question I want to see where it's going in order to avoid intellectualizing the therapy.)*

Jim: Yeah, you're a victim of your training all right—a robot. You can't break loose from the fucking limitations of the world you live in. You claim to understand more, but you don't. You expect me to fit neatly into your sterile, meaningless reality. Forget it. *(Jim is still standing, flipping through the pages of the book he has taken.)*

GAF: Our agreement was that the purpose of this work was to help you to explore and sort out your situation. Any discussion of who I am and where I come from doesn't contribute to that purpose. We have repeatedly agreed on this point. Yet I can see that you persist in avoiding the agreed-upon, free-flowing narration of your thoughts and feelings. So I can only assume that the 'hellbent on destruction' part of you is in charge right now, that you're working toward becoming Nietzsche's 'philosopher of the dangerous', and that martyrdom is your inevitable destiny. The part of you that's driving in this direction is relentlessly opposed to your work here. It cloaks itself in Nietzsche's philosophy of the Antichrist, the chaos of Rimbaud, and the darkness of Kafka. But behind all these ideas are the driving forces of self-hate and an intolerable emptiness. These forces are sending you hurtling you to your death. And the mystical perspectives serve to hide the truth from you. *(I am addressing Jim's inner world in the way that I believe he experiences it.)*

Jim: *(Just stares at me. He is considering my comments. After a few minutes, he responds in a less offensive voice.)* So you . . . you have the answers? You and Sigmund? *(Jim's sarcasm, though not biting, clouds his awareness of the despair he feels. There is a long silence.)* You want me to talk? Want to know what's in my mind huh? I've already told you. Maybe you missed it, Gerald. It's about experience . . . it's Dionysian, taking a full measure of everything, spirit and flesh. No restrictions on our natural instincts. We've been here before, and I'm getting bored. *(Pauses, looks off vacantly)* Can't you dig it, man? Nietzsche's Antichrist, he's . . . totally, totally his own man, totally alone — the defiant one. *(Another long pause. Jim is meandering, his verbalizations a mixture of free associations and fantasies.*) I'm like the shaman, touching the forces and power of other worlds, other . . . existences. *(Another lapse into a reflective silence. After a while, Jim looks up, and for a fleeting moment, flashes a look of unutterable agony. Then nothing. I take note of an instantaneous shudder passing through me, and remain silent. He then rambles on, staring blankly out the window.)* You see, all the groundless worrying about good and evil, right and wrong, they just prevent us from . . . uh . . . being in the true reality. The Antichrist defeats the true evil, the evil of nothingness, the dark nothingness of this reality. The meaningless nothingness. *(Another long pause and again the trance-like appearance.)* I once wrote a poem about . . . uh . . . it was called 'Horse Latitudes.' The Old World Spaniards sailing to the new world would sometimes find themselves stuck in a static atmospheric condition—the doldrums . . . so they would lighten the ship by heaving the cargo over the side. Horses were often the main cargo. I could see them pushing these animals into the sea. Imagine them falling through the air and then struggling to stay afloat. But as their strength gave out, they would sink into the depths, sink . . ever so slowly into the nothingness of the sea. (*Another brief silence, and then he continues.*) So you see, the only solution is to destroy the illusion of this fake reality, to break through to the other reality. Do you see, man, it's all fake . . . all fake. (*Jim turns and looks at some books in a bookcase next to his chair, gets up and scans one title, then another and another until he has read the titles of a dozen or more. He is drawn to A Psychoanalytic Study Of The Myth of Dionysus And Apollo by Helene Deutsch and Object Love And Reality: An Introduction To A Psychoanalytic Theory Of Object Relations by Arnold Modell.*) Are these some of your sacred texts, your guides to reality? Who is Helene Deutsch? (*Opening the book cover, he reads the subtitle.*) "Two variants on the son-mother relationship. The son who saves, the son who kills." What's this bullshit? Who is this chick? If this is what you're reading . . . what a bummer. Is she talking about Dionysus and Apollo in terms of their mothers? Christ, everything with Freud is mother. He was a genius but he had a one track mind. Dionysian mythology had it right on. The only way out of the meaninglessness of his existence . . he senses, and raw, unfettered experience. And what are object relations? This guy Modell . . . does he mean people? Why doesn't he say so? What reality does he mean? You still have nothing to say? *(Jim is still standing, trying to engage me in an intellectual discussion.)*

GAF: Well, I can see how you would be attracted to both Dionysus and Neitzsche's Antichrist-Redeemer. I've been noticing again how you continue to talk about meaninglessness and nothingness.

Jim: Yeah . . . you're on that road again. Why Dionysus? *(Jim is somewhat curious despite his cynicism. He also has hidden hopes that I have a solution for his despair.)*

GAF: Live life to the fullest, gratify the senses, experience everything, and maybe the meaninglessness will become meaningfulness, the nothingness may then become something.

Jim: Yeah, yeah I know. And the Antichrist . . . uh . . . that's where my self-destructive side shows up.

(Jim is sarcastic but he is talking about his beliefs and he is still harboring some hope of rescue from the Dead Zone.)

GAF: Yes, the Antichrist is one of the ways the malevolent forces within you are pulling you toward death. They say, 'accept the chaos, revel in the darkness, embrace death since you cannot escape the nothingness.'

Jim is trying to reject my comments but they touch on what he is experiencing and he becomes stuck. His internal momentum to self-destruct is just slowed by the realization that my observations are speaking to his true feelings and dilemmas. He stares out the window again, appearing to drift into a kind of calm, emotional place. He is in a state similar to a toddler playing in the same room as mom, not interacting with her, but doing his own thing. This state of emotional well being while in the "present-non-interacting-acting other" has been described by the British Analyst W. W. Winnicott as the capacity to be alone, alone together, and is a significant step in a child's development.

The session ends after more discussion of arrangements for future meetings. This session has further revealed the persistent threat to life preserving instincts found in the dead zone.

Jim will come for fourteen more sessions before leaving the Doors and moving to France. The next session is the last one. He is leaving for France in four days.

Session 24.

Jim: *(As expected he is better and worse.)* Well, maybe you've made a few points, Gerald. You're not so bad for who you are. But I'll be glad to get out of here.

GAF: Uh huh. Do you want the names of a few therapists in Paris?

Jim: Yeah, sure. If it makes you feel better. Can't you let it alone? I'm going to be working on my poetry. I'll see what happens. *(Despite his attitude, Jim sounds less certain and even worried. He sits down, his anger not in evidence.)*

GAF: You're vague and noncommittal about this, and I fear that if you don't continue your work with an experienced therapist, you will not do well in Paris.

Jim: Well, your pessimism is encouraging. My life isn't dependent on therapy, or on you, or on anyone. You keep making the same point over and over. Why won't I do well? ? *(Jim's voice still sounds more anxious than angry.)*

GAF: What has changed? You still feel the same confusion about who you are, the same nameless dread that causes you to act self-destructively. The same impulses toward chaos and death. What makes you believe that these forces of despair won't be with you wherever you go?

Jim: Because I have my poetry. That's who I am and it's enough. And Paris is the place. *(Sensing that I'm skeptical of his plan, Jim sits forward, obviously angry.)* What? What? You're pissing me off. Can't you dig it? I'm not like everybody else. Don't measure me by the norms you use for others. I've been different from the beginning.

GAF: Perhaps. But what reason can there be for you to reject the idea of continuing with a therapist except to block your progress toward emotional health?

Jim: Maybe I don't need this bullshit. Maybe I think you're a fucking asshole and I'm wasting my time.

GAF: *(Sitting back in his chair, Jim looks miffed, becomes silent. Jim is desperately trying to maintain his emotional distance. He is doing that now by rejecting me and devaluing the work we have done together.)* Mmm. Perhaps you need to be angry with me and to dismiss the work we've done.

Jim: Oh yeah? Why?

GAF: Because you might be feeling sad at leaving. And anger is easier, a shield against the feeling.

Jim: (*Faint smile, looking away.*) Yeah, sure. Why would I miss this — and having to pay for it, too.

GAF: Because it may be the first time you have felt hope, and found some relief for your confusion and angst. And maybe because you think of me as a friend you'll be leaving. `

Jim: (*Silence. I have touched on Jim's inner experience at this moment and he is now feeling the sadness. But historically he has shown little tolerance for this place in the human heart, and he will soon leave it and me behind as with all his close relationships. For a moment I think I see his eyes become moist, but that quickly passes.*)

Jim: Yeah . . . yeah. Just give me the fucking names if it makes you happy. I told you, you're okay. Maybe you have some interesting ideas. Maybe I'll look up one of these geniuses. (*I hand him a slip with the names of several Parisian analysts.*) Thanks.

Jim Morrison died in Paris of an apparent overdose of heroin. We cannot be certain that his descent into the "knowing void" could have been halted, that a continuation of the psychotherapy constructed in this book would have saved him. The scope of the tragedy of his early death is widened when one considers that, although he sensed that something was wrong, he couldn't have understood the nature of the forces arrayed against him.

Epilogue

This book has been written for all of those who suffer the torment of life in the dead zone. We hope we have provided our readers with a very different understanding of the lives of Janis Joplin and Jim Morrison. We have shown how inaccurate were the many popular explanations of how each died, and how inadequate were the descriptive accounts of their everyday struggles. While we have nothing but superlatives for their biographers and biographies — undertaken with great care as they were by noted authors — we have nonetheless revealed how each external account of the two performers was not able to order the disparate details of their lives into a coherent, causal explanation. As described earlier, the developments in clinical research during the thirty or so years since Janis and Jim died have provided us with a very useful framework within which to explain the personality disorders that took their lives.

We think, however, that our analysis here may offer readers more than a very revealing answer to the question, "What was wrong with them?" The insights into the lives of Janis and Jim that we have provided are, we think, interesting enough, especially to those who retain a strong interest in their music and personalities. But we believe these insights have broader applications to many, many others in our society who suffer from the various types of borderline disorders. So, in a sense, our account of these two famous borderline personalities may assist not only other clinicians and psychotherapists to recognize patients so afflicted, but might also help to establish a line between the social and the psychological, between the easy acceptance of individual idiosyncracies and the common recognition of emotional imbalance.

Our work here may thus help a larger audience—one less familiar with the complications of personality disorders—to distinguish merely eccentric, flashy, and indecent behaviors from those behaviors that are suggestive of serious emotional illness. As we cast our gaze backward onto the tumultuous decade of the 1960s, we cannot but notice the then prevailing popular tendencies to legitimate the odd and bizarre, the "hyper" and the "hipper," the excessive and obsessive. We heard the disciples of Timothy Leary urging us to tune out and turn on, to "do your own thing," to join the revolution and "seize the time." It is not our intention to quarrel with those who espoused such messages, nor to demonize them. Rather we chose to disclose the relationship that existed between the very popular socio-political thematics that characterized the 60s, widely embraced as they were by those who idolized Janis and Jim, and the easy acceptance of the self-destructive behaviors for which Janis and Jim were so well known.

To frame this differently, to a significant extent, the many outrageous behaviors exhibited by Janis and Jim were legitimated by the veneer of respectability that was supported by those sympathetic to countercultural expressions prevalent during the 60s. Making this claim does not undercut the role that other forces and factors may have played in the adulation of behaviors that proved so lethal to Janis and Jim.

Thus, for example, the fact that they were two very talented, highly artistic and very successful performers and musicians also helped to deflect substantial criticisms of their "antics" on stage, which were as likely to be confused with sophisticated artistic merit as to have been associated with emotional disturbance. That many fans often associated the two with "anti-establishment" political positions, with a profound recognition of the alienative effects of post-industrial capitalism, with the consequences of an unpopular and ill-fated Southeast Asian war, could understandably have deflected anyone from noticing what we might easily observe today to be severe emotional distress. Clinical research was not yet ready to identify and treat the symptoms of their emotional conflicts and dread, while the great socio-political turmoil of the decade had many mesmerized by the power and energy of their performances. Thus, Janis and Jim performed themselves to death, embraced by their awe-struck fans who were already inclined to see only the mystical, the raucous, and the dazzle.

Of course, this work has had the benefit of retrospect, of a more informed backward glance at the 60's through the prism of modern psychiatry and psychology. We hope that this work will help our readers disentangle the forces in play that led to the tragic deaths of Janis and Jim.

Appendix I

DSM-IV Criteria For Borderline Personality Disorder

A pervasive pattern of instability of interpersonal relationships, self-image, and affects, and marked impulsivity beginning by early adulthood and present in a variety of contexts, as indicated by five (or more) of the following

1. frantic efforts to avoid real or imagined abandonment.
Note: Does not include suicidal or self-mutilating behavior covered in Criterion 5.

2. a pattern of unstable and intense interpersonal relationships characterized by alternating between extremes of idealization and devaluation.

3. identity disturbance: markedly and persistently unstable self-image or sense of self.

4. impulsivity in at least two areas that are potentially self-damaging (e.g., spending, sex, substance abuse, reckless driving, binge eating).
Note: Does not include suicidal or self-mutilating behavior covered in Criterion 5.

5. recurrent suicidal behavior, or threats, or self-mutilating behavior.

6. affective instability due to a marked reactivity of mood (e.g., intense episodic dysphoria, irritability, or

anxiety usually lasting a few hours and only rarely more than a few days.

7. chronic feelings of emptiness.

8. Inappropriate intense anger or difficulty controlling anger (e.g., frequent displays of temper, constant anger, recurrent physical fights).

9. transient, stress-related paranoid ideation or severe dissociative symptoms.

Appendix II

DSM-IV Criteria for Major Depressive Episode

A. Five (or more) of the following symptoms have been present during the same 2-week period and represent a change from previous functioning; at least one of the symptoms is either (1) depressed mood or (2) loss of interest or pleasure.
Note: Do not include symptoms that are clearly due to a general medical condition, or mood-incongruent delusions or hallucinations.

1. depressed mood most of the day, nearly every day, as indicated by either subjective report (e.g., feels sad or empty) or observation made by others (e.g., appears tearful).
Note: In children and adolescents, can be irritable mood.

2. markedly diminished interest or pleasure in all, or almost all, activities most of the day, nearly every day (as indicated by either subjective account or observation made by others)

3. significant weight loss when not dieting or weight gain (e.g., a change of more than 5% of body weight in a month), or decrease or increase in appetite nearly every day. Note: In children, consider failure to make expected weight gains.

4. insomnia or hypersomnia nearly every day.

5. psychomotor agitation or retardation nearly every

day (observable by others, not merely subjective feelings of restlessness or being slowed down).

6. fatigue or loss of energy nearly every day

7. feelings of worthlessness or excessive or inappropriate guilt (which may be delusional) nearly every day (not merely self-reproach or guilt about being sick).

8. diminished ability to think or concentrate, or indecisiveness, nearly every day (either by subjective account or as observed by others).

9. recurrent thoughts of death (not just fear of dying), recurrent suicidal ideation without a specific plan, or a suicide attempt or a specific plan for committing suicide.

Bibliography

Clinical Literature

Deutsch H: "Some Forms of Emotional Disturbance and Their Relationship to Schizophrenia." *Psychoanalytic Quarterly*, 11:301-321.

Diagnostic and Statistical Manual of Mental Disorders (fourth edition). Washington: The American Psychiatric Association, 1994 [DSM IV]

Grinker, R. R., Sr., Werble, B., & Drye, R. C. (1968), *The Borderline Syndrome.* New York: Basic Books.

Grotstein, J. S., Solomon, M. F. & Lang, J. A. (1987) *The Borderline Patient: Emerging Concepts in Diagnosis, Psychodynamics, and Treatment.* Vols. I & II, Hillsdale, New Jersey: Analytic Press.

Gunderson J. (1977) *"Characteristics of Borderlines."* In *Borderline Personality Disorders*, ed. P. Hartocollis. New York: International Universities Press, pp. 173-192.

Gunderson, J. (1982), "Empirical Studies of the Borderline Diagnosis." In *Psychiatry* 1982: Annual Review, ed. L. Grinspoon. Amer. Psychiat. Press, pp. 415-436.

Gunderson, J. & Kolb, J. (1978), "Discriminating Features of Borderline Patients." *Amer. J. Psychiat.*, 135(7):792-796.

Gunderson, J. & Singer, M. T. (1975) "Defining

Borderline Patients: An Overview. *American Journal of Psychiatry*, 132:1-10.

Kernberg O. (1967) "Borderline Personality Organization." *Journal of the American Psychoanalysis Association* 15:641-685.

Kernberg O. (1976) "Technical Considerations in the Treatment of Borderline Personality Organization." *Journal of the American Psychoanalysis Asso*ciation 24:795-829.

Kernberg O. (1975) *Borderline Conditions and Pathological Narcissism.* New York: Jason Aronson.

Kernberg O. (1984) *Severe Personality Disorders:* Psychotherapeutic Strategies. New Haven: Yale University Press.

Meissner, W. (1984) *The Borderline Sprectrum.* New York: Jason Aronson.

Perry, J. C., & Klerman, G. L. (1978) "The Borderline Patient." *Archives of General. Psychiatry.*, 35:141-150.

Winnicott D W: (1965) *The Maturational Processes and the Facilitating Environment.* New York: International Universities Press.

Janis Joplin

Amburn, E. (1992) *Pearl: The Obsessions and Passions of Janis Joplin.* New York: Warner Books.

Caserta, Peggy. (1973) *Going Down With Janis,* as told to Don Knapp. New York: Dell.

Freidman, Myra. (1992)   *Buried Alive.* New York: Harmony Books.

Joplin, Laura. (1992) *Love, Janis.* New York: Villard Books.

Film: *Janis, The Way She Was.* (1974 documentary), MCA Home Video 80080.

Jim Morrison

Densmore, John. (1990) *Riders on the Storm.* New York: Delacorte Press.

Hopkins, Jerry & Sugarman, Danny. (1980) *No One Here Gets Out Alive.* New York: Warner Books.

Kennealy, Patricia. (1992) *Strange Days: My Life With and Without Jim Morrison.* New York: Dutton.

Morrison, Jim. (1970) *The Lords and the New Creatures.* New York: Simon & Schuster.

---------- (1988) *Wilderness.* New York: Villard Books

---------- (1990) *The American Night.* New York: Villard Books.

Riordan, James & Prochnicky, Jerry. (1991) *Break on Through: The Life and Death of Jim Morrison.* New York: William Morrow.

ISBN 155212378-2